INSTANT PAIN RELIEF

How Neural/Fascial Therapy Offers Rapid Therapeutic Response with Complete Correction of Chronic Pain

by

William J. Faber, D.O.

Practicing Doctor of Osteopathic Medicine

Founder and Medical Director

MILWAUKEE PAIN CLINIC

AND METABOLIC RESEARCH CENTER

Milwaukee, Wisconsin

and

Morton Walker, D.P.M.

Medical Journalist and Editorial Director

FREELANCE COMMUNICATIONS

Stamford, Connecticut

Biological Publications Milwaukee, Wisconsin

June 1991

ISBN: 1-879361-00-0
Library of Congress Catalog Number: 90-84565

TABLE OF CONTENTS

ABOUT THE AUTHORS

WILLIAM J. FABER, D.O., a biology and chemistry graduate of Drake University and the University of Health Sciences, College of Osteopathic Medicine, is board certified in Pain Management Specialties and Biological Reconstructive Therapy by the American Academy of Neurological and Orthopaedic Surgeons. In 1989, he was presented with "The Best Paper of the Year" award from the American Academy of Neurological and Orthopaedic Surgeons for his published scholarly paper, "German Neural-Fascial Therapy." In much greater depth but written in easier-to-understand language, the information in that paper has been reproduced in this book.

Periodically throughout each year, Dr. Faber teaches neural-fascial therapy and reconstructive therapy to physicians in preceptorship programs. They arrive from all over the United States and from foreign nations to learn from him the procedure's intricate technique of application.

Dr. Faber is a founding member of the Institutional Review Board of the Great Lakes Association of Clinical Medicine. Also he is a member of the board of directors of the American Academy of Biological Dentistry.

Dr. Faber has appeared on over 150 radio and television shows throughout North America, and he lectures on health problems to lay and professional audiences extensively. He is in the process of writing additional books and scripts for various audio-video productions. For instance, he

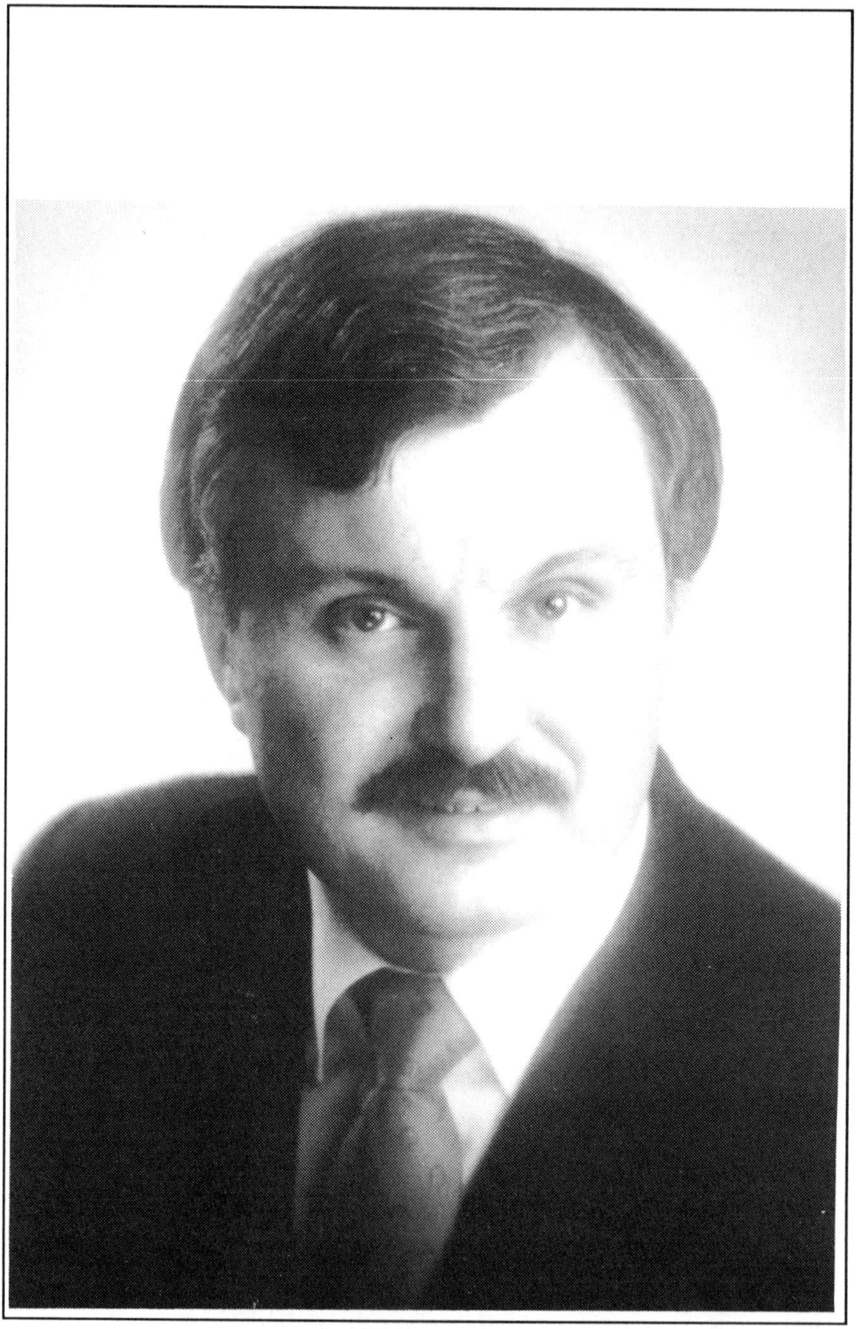

William J. Faber D.O.
F.A.A.N.O.S.
Physician, Researcher, Teacher

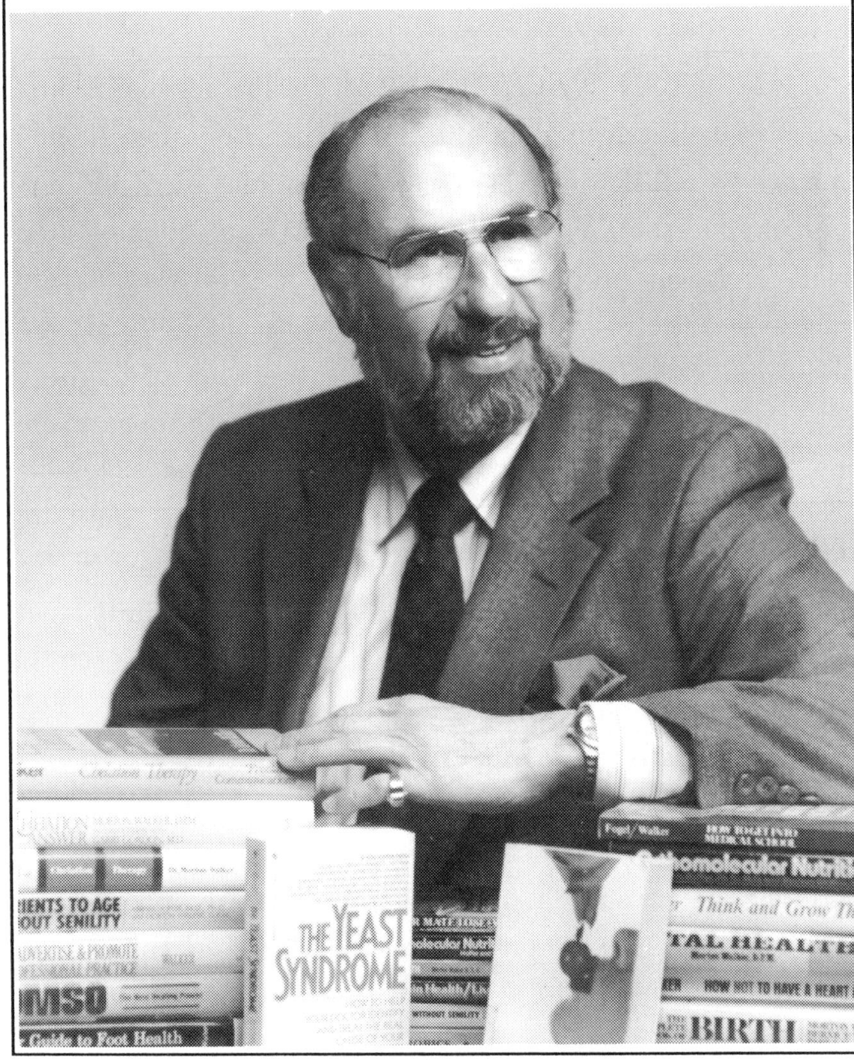

Morton Walker D.P.M.
Medical journalist, Author, Lecturer

is coauthor with Dr. Morton Walker of Pain, Pain Go Away (Ishi Press International, 1990, a $12.95 trade paperback). Dr. Faber's health care articles have appeared in more than twenty consumer magazines and scientific journals. He is listed in Who's Who in the Midwest and Who's Who of Emerging Leaders.

****

MORTON WALKER, D.P.M., a former practicing doctor of podiatric medicine, changed his profession in 1969 to work as a fulltime, freelance, professional medical journalist and author. To his credit Dr. Walker has 50 published books and over 1400 published clinical journal articles and magazine articles on all aspects of wholistic medicine, orthomolecular nutrition, and alternative methods of healing. Eight of his bestsellers each have hundreds of thousands of copies in print. By educating several million readers, he is acclaimed for being responsible for improving the quality of their lives and increasing the average person's longevity. He receives over a dozen telephone calls and letters daily from fans around the globe who advise him of how lifestyle is better for them because of what he has written.

Health professional and journalism organizations have recognized Dr. Walker's excellence by awarding him with 22 gold, silver, and bronze medals and two plaques. He received them from the American College of Advancement in Medicine, the Institute of Preventive Medicine, the American Business Press, the American Podiatry Association, and The Journal of Current Podiatric Medicine.

Dr. Walker appears regularly before the public and on

media, so far in more than 1200 radio, television, and press interviews. He lectures on a broad range of health subjects throughout the United States and around the world. He has delivered talks in 18 foreign countries on complementary medicine and other health subjects. Information comes to him by means of his search of the medical literature and his interviews of health professionals who are on the cutting edge of new advances in medicine.

Out of just such interviews, Dr. Faber and Dr. Walker formed an alliance that has them collaborating on a number of public communication projects. Instant Pain Relief is their second co-authored book, and a third one is in production.

****

DISCLAIMER

This book has been written and published strictly for informational purposes, and in no way should it be used as a substitute for your own physician's advice.

While William J. Faber, D.O. and Morton Walker, D.P.M., are collaborating here as co-authors, Dr. Faber is the physician expert on instant pain relief and Dr. Walker is the medical journalist reporting on such health care information.

You should not consider educational material in this book to be the practice of medicine, although almost all the facts have come from the files, publications, and personal interviews of informed physicians who diagnose and treat with neural/fascial therapy and/or their patients who have suffered from chronic pain syndromes. Moreover, clinical journal articles, popular magazine articles, material from published books, lecture presentations, audiotapes, case reports, anecdotes, testimonials, patient histories, and other information have been utilized to educate our readers.

If you, as a potential user of knowledge received from these pages, require opinions, diagnoses, treatments, therapeutic advice, correction of your lifestyle, or any other aid relating to your health, it is recommended that you consult either Dr. Faber, the other physicians contributing to this book, or your own medical expert on the chronic pain syndrome that you face. A list of such neural/fascial therapy experts is appended to this book.

These statements are to be considered disclaimers of responsibility for anything published here. The co-authors provide the information in this book with the understanding that you may act on it at your own risk and also with full knowledge that health professionals should first be consulted and that their specific advice for you should be considered before anything read here.

ACKNOWLEDGEMENTS

Special recognition is deserving of the staff of the Milwaukee Pain Clinic and Metabolic Research Center in Milwaukee, Wisconsin. These efficient, capable, and energetic workers performed their duties professionally and with dynamism. These six effectual people include Barbara Rothe, Rita Hirsch, Kathy Rogers, Helen Jackson, Chandra Lynk, and Ginny Laughlin. Their attention to the many aspects of putting this book together is deeply appreciated.

Also held in deep respect are the patients who shared their stories, photographs, and medical data. Some have traveled great distances to find relief. Their contributions allow myriad others who are suffering to find their own health havens away from the clutches of pain and disability.

Special consideration is expressed to Dr. Morton Walker of Stamford, Connecticut who put in extra effort to relay the biological science of neural-fascial therapy in clear, concise language. His skill as a writer highly educates the health consumer. Dr. Walker's exceptional talents are displayed on each page of this book.

Thanks are expressed to Leszek Zielinski of Artex Press in Stevens Point, Wisconsin who supervised the text's typesetting and printing.

Also acknowledged are the expertise of M.G.I. Graphics of Milwaukee, Wisconsin, the Medical College of Wisconsin Library Research Staff, and artist Richard Marvin Voigt for technical and creative assistance.

PREFACE

Pain is one of life's paradoxes: on one hand, it's a universal phenomenon that everyone experiences at least occasionally during life. Yet it's so personal and private that each person's experience is unique. The sufferer himself is the only true expert on his pain.

In its many forms, ranging from sharp stabs to dull aches, pain demands attention—sometimes to the exclusion of all other considerations. The word itself derives from the Greek word for <u>penalty</u>, suggesting an ancient perception of pain as a price we pay for living.

Of course, pain is not designed as random punishment. Rather, it's a primal warning system that protects against injury and encourages immobilization during healing. Although acute pain can be excruciating, it's usually both transient and purposeful. It's something else, too, when the pain becomes chronic. Then it loses obvious meaning and threatens well-being. Usually chronic pain is a signal of internal dysfunction that something has gone awry with a singular segment of the body, perhaps only a few cellular elements or a major portion of the physiologic system.

Despite pain's universality, it has been an incompletely understood phenomenon that is usually discussed in terms of theory, not fact. Physiology and perception have been so tightly intertwined that distinguishing one element from the other is sometimes impossible. One result of society's confusion is that pain—whether acute or chronic—has often been inadequately managed, to the detriment of the pain victim.

All that confusion is changing to enlightenment now that neural/fascial therapy has come upon the scene. The concepts of this treatment's inventors, the Huneke brothers, two German physicians, now deceased, explain a great deal about the cause and character of chronic pain and physical dysfunction.

Acute Pain Versus Chronic Pain

Although some may be inclined to think of chronic pain as an extension of acute pain, the two pain types differ significantly in many ways. Let us look at them:

By definition, acute pain lasts less than six months; chronic pain, more than six months.

Acute pain usually is highly localized; chronic pain probably is poorly localized. The character of acute pain usually has it feeling sharp, perhaps radiating, and generally arising from an acute injury or disease process, and it passes quickly.

Chronic pain often is dull, aching, diffuse, constant, nagging, and intractable. Chronic pain may be associated with chronic pathology, or it may persist after recovery from a disease or injury.

Acute pain is associated with autonomic nervous system response including increased blood pressure, increased heart rate, sweating, pallor, widening of the eyes' pupils, restlessness, grimacing facial expression, and anxiety. Chronic pain may or may not have autonomic nervous system response, but the patient feels exhausted, and acts listless, depressed, and withdrawn.

A person experiencing acute pain often expects medical intervention to relieve it.

The individual suffering from chronic pain anticipates only that medical intervention may reduce the pain, but he or she also believes that its presence and chronicity will continue. Such a common belief was valid before the advent of neural/fascial therapy, but now rapid therapeutic response is a common occurrence when this new/old treatment is administered by open-minded, well-trained, and skilled biologic physicians.

Because chronic pain has become America's most common, expensive, and debilitating disorder, and because too many doctors and pain sufferers know surprisingly little about the causes of pain and the wide variety of treatments that are available today, our book had to be written, must be read, and demands a reaction to the new information it imparts. We have not lightly chosen Instant Pain Relief as its title. This title implies a promise that readily is kept when action is taken according to our text's presentations, descriptions, and directions.

It is a comprehensive guide that provides the pain victim with lasting alleviation of discomfort. The authors have attempted to write in an encouraging, understandable, and readable style so as to explain why you hurt, what your pain means, and how to quickly get permanent pain relief.

We hope you do agree that our attempts have been successful.

Each day around the world, millions of people suffer pain and loss of motion in joints, fingers, knees, ankles, wrists, internal organs, and other body parts as a result of contractures and spasm. They are put into braces, physical supports, crutches, exercises, medications, and emotional support groups. All this does not correct the problems they face because the treatments fail to correct the causes of the problems.

If a traditionally-practicing allopathic physician chooses to treat diseases or illnesses, the textbooks—like cookbooks—state to give this drug or do that surgery. For the thinking person a few fair questions would be: If you have an infection does this mean you are suffering from a shortage of antibiotics or some other manufactured substance? If surgery is recommended, does this mean you have an extra part or you will do better with less or some rearranged body parts?

We can send men to the moon and explore the solar system but so often medical meccas tell seeking people that they will "just have to learn to live with pain and disability." Such a statement is a blatant falsehood now that we have neural/fascial therapy to offer the afflicted.

This book deals with a therapy which is known to provide instant relief of pain, increased motion, and return of function for problems not able to be aided by any other method. The therapy is known as new/old German neural/fascial therapy: new because it's likely that you are learning about it for the first time; old because it was developed in Germany in 1925 and has been actively practiced in Europe since 1928. The treatment is used for pain problems ranging literally from head to toe. The results of pain relief become permanent when all the problems of ill-health are corrected. Neural/fascial therapy is effective in correcting them.

While every individual case history presented by us is true and about a real person, pseudonyms are employed because of requirements of many of the state medical societies. The information in this book comes from literature searches and other research done by co-author Morton Walker, D.P.M. and from patient interviews he conducted. The case reports, patient contacts, and the scientific basis for neural/fascial pain elimination have been supplied by William J. Faber, D.O. and his colleagues. A few certain doctors have taken training in the techniques of joint reconstruction, participate in preceptorships, and attend seminars on the subject so as to exchange new information with each other.

The primary instruments of patient repair utilized for neural/fascial therapeutic response are the hypodermic needle and syringe. No other device delivers such precise medicine and corrective therapy with such minimum trauma to a human being than the hypodermic needle. No other device has relieved more pain and saved more lives than the hypodermic needle. Our intent as authors is to make the explanation about this new/old German injection method so clear and illustrative of its benefits that you will feel yourself compelled to give it a try if you are the victim of any kind of discomfort at all.

We have some concluding bits of philosophical advice as it relates to improving health, ridding yourself of pain, and feeling happy:

Watch your thoughts, they become words.
Watch your words, they become actions.
Watch your actions, they become habits.
Watch your habits, they become character.
Watch your character, it becomes your destiny.
The choice is yours!

Everything—all aspects of life—follow this rule: You get nothing for nothing, but do receive a tit for a tat!

What are you doing to build your health? Are you working at any structural reconstruction, using detoxification techniques, performing regular exercises, stabilizing your emotions, eating natural whole foods, drinking distilled or reverse osmosis water, or learning a lifestyle of total wellness?

Remember to invest in yourself. There are no trade-ins. Everyone gets what he or she deserves.

What do you want? The choice is yours!

Remember also that desire and knowledge are the initial steps toward making that choice, while action and perseverance are the final steps to achieving health or any other kind of success.

Wishing you the best in health and all things, we are

— William J. Faber, D.O., Milwaukee, Wisconsin

— Morton Walker, D.P.M., Stamford, Connecticut

August 1, 1990

FOREWORD

It was shortly after I opened the first Veramed Cancer Clinic that I learned a valuable lesson about pain and how amazingly effective neural/fascial therapy can be. Thirty-four-year-old Fraulein Elsa Maria von Betrand, a recurrently painful breast cancer patient, effectively taught me that important lesson.

Elsa had undergone mastectomy—her left breast was removed two years earlier. Following surgery, she quickly received four months of followup with traditional chemotherapy to prevent any recurrence of this deadly disease in the other breast. From her surgeons she heard that awful cliché and invariable lie, "We got it all!" Twenty months later new tumorous growths appeared directly on her healed surgical site and also under the left armpit.

Elsa wanted no repeat of the typically severe side effects that accompany chemotherapy. A different approach was required, and she eventually heard of the nontoxic biological methods which are emphasized at my Veramed Cancer Clinic in Nussdorf, West Germany. She was anxious to start her personalized, inpatient, intensive biological program. The nutrition plan, regional hyperthermia, oxygen/ozone treatment, colon cleansing, lymphatic drainage, vitamins and minerals, herbs, enzymes, mind training, and immunostimulation that make up nontoxic, unconventional cancer treatment caused a shrinkage of her tumors to nothing. My staff of physicians and I could find no trace of them at all by the end of her course of therapy.

Elsa expressed happiness that she was out of danger from breast cancer; yet, she remained in a state of discomfort. She was experiencing a lack of motion at the left shoulder, felt as if her skin was being tugged tightly, had a certain sensation that pulling downward was taking place, and was suffering with persistent pain around the two-year-old mastectomy scar. To any medical observer, the slightly pink scar looked well-healed with no irregularities seemingly present, but Elsa complained of general discomfort.

I saw Elsa's disappointment that her pain and dysfunction remained an integral part of her life; consequently, I suggested neural/fascial therapy injections into the scar. She agreed. No sooner had I placed the last milliliter of procaine anesthetic into the surgical site than I witnessed color change and new vitality coming over Elsa's face and body. She rose from the treatment table, raised her arm up and down several times, and a light shone in her eyes that said she had reached her goal of health and happiness. The patient reported that pain had gone along with the feelings of skin tugging and pulling.

For me, this experience of a patient's joy has since become commonplace. The incident with Elsa, while one of the first I witnessed from utilizing neural/fascial therapy, is only one small example of how such a simple, local injection can bring about dramatic effects of ease and comfort for people in pain.

As a result of their taking the original German concepts of the Drs. Huneke, then applying osteopathic structural principles and the laws of physics, next furnishing a broader comprehension and usage of this new/old neural/fascial therapy, and finally bringing the message of hope and healing to readers around the world, this book's authors, Dr. William J. Faber and Dr. Morton Walker, deserve much appreciation and, indeed, our highest award of gratitude. Their book is superb scientific writing and very easy reading that is concise and readily followed.

Assuredly Dr. Faber knew what he was doing when he prevailed upon Dr. Walker to lay out the modified science of neural/fascial therapy so as to be readily accepted by the public and open-minded health care professionals, alike.

In turn, Dr. Walker recognized just as well that Dr. Faber provides a life-preserving procedure which demands greater exposure than merely what is available in the usual one-to-one relationship of a small treatment room.

Teamed together in Instant Pain Relief, the co-authors are aiding all of us to improve the quality of our lives. Along with a flowing and comprehensive text, the illustrations and actual photographs furnished are graphic and precise. Here we have a presentation in depth showing the significance of new/old German neural/fascial therapy. Drs. Walker and Faber have personally offered me insightful perspectives despite my having employed this pain-relieving treatment method for over 15 years.

By far the greatest thanks, of course, will come from millions of patients all over the Western industrialized world who are administered neural/fascial therapy by knowledgeable and skillful doctors. These patients are bound to become more productive from the essential information laid out in Instant Pain Relief. The whole of society will benefit.

Too bad that the neural/fascial technique of eliminating pain does not get taught in any medical schools and residency programs. However, from acting on the information imparted by this text, all those afflicted who seek freedom from suffering, plus the health professionals wishing to render correction for that silent assailant we refer to as pain, this book becomes a valuable tool.

I anticipate that Instant Pain Relief will be reprinted in German and other languages so that this masterful work of Dr. Faber and Dr. Walker can be utilized by all people around the globe who need the rapid therapeutic response furnished by neural/fascial therapy.

—Professor of Medicine Frederich R. Douwes, M.D.,
Medical Director of the Veramed Cancer Clinics,
Nussdorf, The Federal Republic of Germany
August 1, 1990

Introduction

THE SILENT ASSAILANT

Pain, as Dr. Frederich Douwes implied in his foreword, is a silent assailant that cannot be defined, except by you when you feel it.

Taking your pain to some doctors is like describing the Mona Lisa to a blind man in a language neither of you understands. You find it difficult to put a description of your pain into words; an unfeeling doctor finds it hard to comprehend and interpret the pain because he or she doesn't know precisely what your words mean to you. Being the silent assailant, pain has no method of measurement, no clinical or laboratory readings to show the extent of how much you hurt.

Numbers of patients have been ill-treated by a few doctors who dismiss their real but chronic pain as "imaginary" and send them to psychiatrists. Others may contemptuously set the victim's continuous sensations of discomfort aside by declaring, "You must have a low threshold," whatever "threshold" means. The silent assailant remains known only to the sufferer and unmeasurable by others. So, it's not uncommon for a person in pain to come to the conclusion that he or she must live with it. As indicated from the information that follows, such a conclusion is erroneous!

This book is about permanently overcoming

chronic pain—not just coping with it. You don't have to live with pain as an ongoing part of your everyday existence.

To get closer to the source and solving of your pain problem, answers to questions often need to be given to the doctor—Where does it hurt? How long has the pain been troubling you? What does it feel like? Does the pain change when you move? Does it wake you up at night? Is your pain related to some incident in the past that left you with a lasting effect?1

The Lasting Effect of Dental Trauma

In Chicago, cocktail waitress Janet Wilson, age 38, had been suffering with facial pain and swelling on the right side of her face for nine years. The pain would be excruciating at times requiring her to lose the ability to function and thus leave work. This happened often enough that she lost jobs and found new employment with eight different establishments during this extended period of time. Her skill at filling drink orders was such that she seldom had difficulty finding a replacement job. Still, Janet recognized that her situation could not continue in the same way indefinitely. The pain and edema surrounding her upper jaw was getting her down—causing anxiety and depression.

She felt pain behind her right ear, alongside the right jaw, at the back of her skull, and in multiple areas of the neck. To be sure, it wasn't your standard tension headache. She visited many different health professionals: an optometrist, two dentists, a psychologist, an ear, nose, and throat specialist, a chiropractor, and some other medical practitioners, but without finding the permanent help she required so badly. Furthermore, the waitress sought other opinions among her relatives and friends, as well, rather than taking strong pain pills and learning merely to live with the pain.

Unfortunately, various dental and medical examinations never turned up the source of her trouble until she walked into the Milwaukee Pain Clinic and Metabolic Reseach Center for a consultation with its medical director, Dr. William J. Faber.

The doctor's physical examination, including a good look into her oral cavity, revealed that Janet possessed a lower right gum area that appeared irregular and was exquisitely tender to the touch. On being questioned, the patient recalled a wisdom tooth removal approximately ten year prior to the onset of her chronic facial and head pains. Following additional clinical tests, the source of difficulty for Janet Wilson became obvious to Dr. Faber.

The dental scar area at the site from which her wisdom tooth had been removed ten years before was too tight. It was pulling on nerves so as to bring on chronic pain and soft tissue swelling around the jaw which radiated to the head. She needed corrective neural/fascial injections, Dr. Faber explained, and the patient agreed to receiving them.

Immediate improvement occurred for Janet with just the first application of a painless injection procedure. She had instant pain relief that lasted half-a-day. Followup treatments, however, brought much more lasting relief, until repeated application of neural/fascial therapy made the comfort permanent. The scar area physically improved in appearance as her tenderness resolved with the loosening corrective injections. Adjunctively, Janet's neck was given reconstructive therapy (see Pain, Pain Go Away by William J. Faber, D.O. and Morton Walker, D.P.M., 1990, Ishi Press International, 330 pages, $12.95) because it was unstable. Her wobbly neck responded with increased firmness, less neck ligamentous fatigue, and the disappearance of pain in the neck joints altogether.

Combining neural/fascial therapy and reconstructive therapy, today Janet Wilson's facial, head, and neck pain and swelling have completely disappeared. It is two years now, and while Janet has taken these injection procedures to correct other uncomfortable body parts, it's not necessary to administer them to the areas that initially brought her to the Milwaukee Pain Clinic.

Impulses that Carry Pain

Your entire neurological system is made up of millions of nerve fibers, which run like an unimaginably complicated highway system from the tips of your fingers and toes to the control center in the brain. The main highway runs up through the spinal column in bundles of nerve fibers that come together with the brain in its stem and that part of the brain called the thalamus. It's along these neurological highways that pain messages pass.

But also along these highways are billions of microscopic interchanges that must receive adequate amounts of chemical substances we derive from our foods if we expect them to work efficiently. This is why specific nutritious foods are so crucial to how you feel and function. Part of neural/fascial therapy includes detoxification of body wastes and nutrient feeding of the body cells to have you in homeostasis (all systems working at peak performance). Detoxification and good nutrition have a direct effect on the brain because they are needed for preventing blockage and for chemical conversions to keep the neurological freeways moving.

Specialized nerve cells, called neurons, carry messages to and from the brain. The neurons originate in receptors, which are specialized nerve endings designed to pick up stimuli from the outside environment such as temperature and pressure. A certain pattern of reception by a set of specialized receptors interprets some sensations as "pain". This message is then carried through the neurons in the form of electrochemical impulses. Many atoms in the body carry an electrical charge. These atoms are called ions and their movement accounts for the body's electrical "current" known as nerve impulses. The end destination for many of the impulses carried by the neurons is the brain, where the sensation of pain is identified and localized. The impulses traverse breaks or small chasms in the nerve chain called synapses, which are bathed in interstitial fluid.

In order for a message to traverse each chasm a substance called a neurotransmitter must be present. Neurotransmitters are complex molecular chemicals such tylcholine, norepinephrine, and serotonin. The quality of your nutrition from which these neurotransmitters are made determines how well such substances do their job of nerve impulse transmission.

Remembering the Sources of Pain

Nerve impulses begin in the receptor's specialized endings. They travel electrochemically along the neuron, across the chasms or breaks between neurons and eventually end in the spinal cord along tracts to the brain. In the brain, the impulses pass through various areas to the thalamus where pain is recognized, and then it goes on to localizing receptors.

In the brain, as well, the messages are acted on by impulses from the five senses, from depression circuits, and from memory traces called engrams, of previous pain experiences. These engrams are memories of how pain affected you in the past. The "color" of pain is altered by these engrams and by expectations of what the pain should be like. Once you have a trauma resulting in pain, even if it occurred to you under general anesthesia or in coma, it gets recorded, and you always hold its memory in your subconscious. In effect, you always remember the sources of pain.

This memory factor for pain is important to know because erasing such a memory of pain from previous trauma, present injury, chronic illness, tightly-pulling scars, or other remote sources, as we shall see in Chapter One, is partly the way neural/fascial therapy works.

Chapter One

THE PHYSICS OF PAIN AND ILLNESS

An East Texas logger and truck driver, Geoffrey Watson, 48 years old, found his way to the office of physician and surgeon John L. Sessions, D.O., of Kirbyville, Texas. The man had a pathetic history which he revealed to Dr. Sessions.

For seven years the unfortunate fellow had been suffering from severe symptoms of reflex sympathetic dystrophy in his left arm and shoulder. Geoffrey was feeling sharp and stabbing pains of a known origin in his neuromuscular system on the left side of the upper body. He explained that there had been a major injury to his left shoulder area due to an auto-truck accident with five attempted operative repairs over the intervening years. The injuries and postsurgical effects seemed to heal uneventfully but then he was left with intermittent excrutiating pain. At first the pain appeared just sporadically and for short periods; later it remained as a chronic source of physical disability and mental stress.

As observed by the physician and surgeon, an inability to move his limb because of this pain had caused Geoffrey's left arm and shoulder muscles to weaken and waste away to about one-half their original bulk. Comparing it to the right arm, Dr. Sessions saw that the patient's left arm looked shrunken. No longer could he work as a logger by sawing wood or swinging an axe. Geoffrey found that his left arm was almost useless, and he was only able to retain the trucker's part of his job by shifting truck gears with his right hand while he barely held the steering wheel steady with his left.

Actually, Geoffrey had sustained a few close calls with near-collisions of his log-filled truck because of a limited wheel-turning ability. He was a menace on the road, and the poor trucker knew it. Pain for him was so bad that the patient considered suicide to end it all. During that interval when he was making legal, financial, social, and other preparations to kill himself, he happened to learn from neighbors of Dr. Sessions' success with eliminating the very type of pain from which Geoffrey suffered.

Over the course of two months, Dr. Sessions administered eleven series of neuro/fascial therapy injections to Geoffrey Watson. The patient felt comforted by them from the very first and improved more with each visit for the next series. The eleventh injection series saw him made totally painfree. Today, three years after his first treatment visit, the man remains free of any discomfort, but he still visits the physician every six to eight months for some booster neuro/fascial therapy. He has gone back to the full duties of logging and trucking.

The Elements of Imbalance of Geoffrey Watson

The difficulty experienced by the patient of John L. Sessions, D.O. exemplifies (see illustration #1 and illustra-

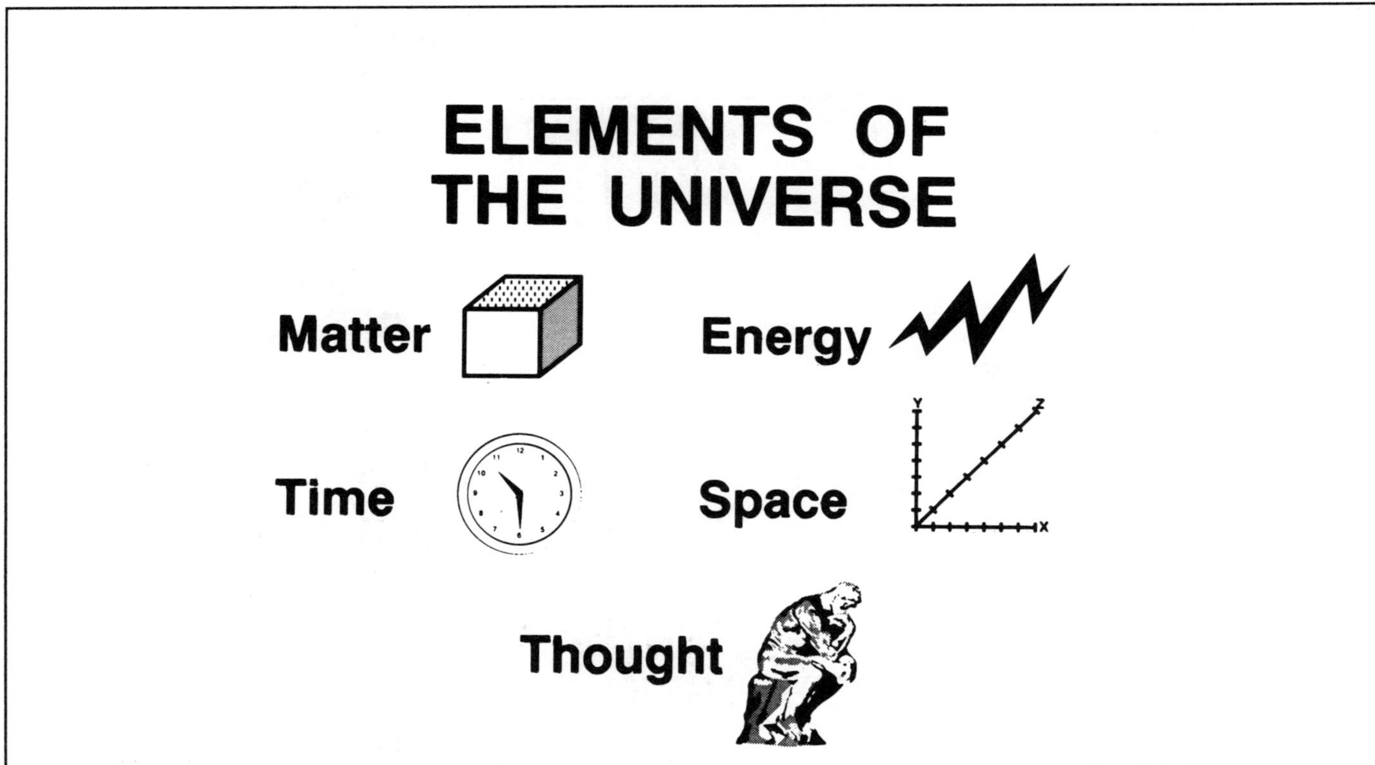

Illustration #1 — All things consist of variable amounts of matter, energy, time, space and thought.

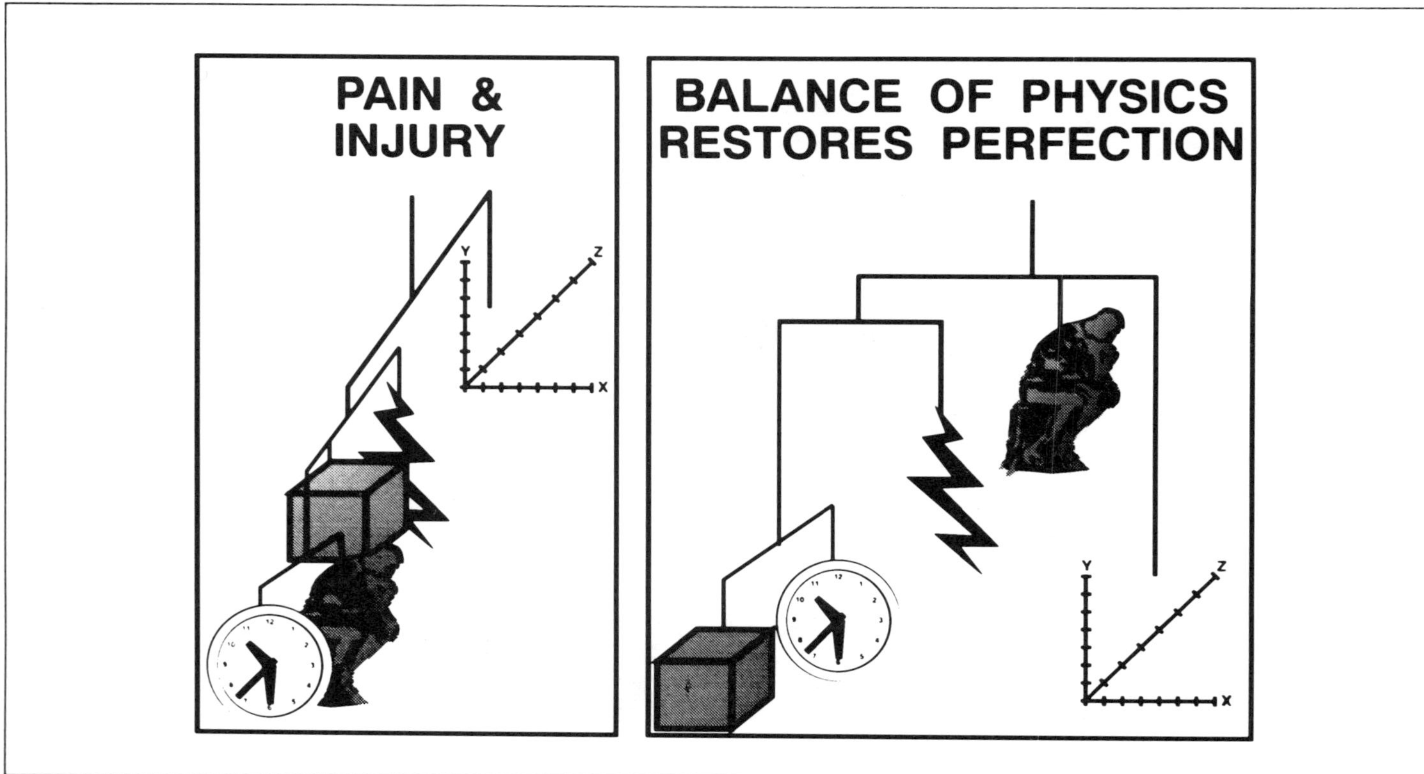

Illustration #2 — Pain and injury are results of imbalances of matter, energy, space, time and thought. Correction involves restoring the balance of these physical elements.

tion #2) broader problems therapists are called upon to solve which relate to physical-medical concepts. The question requiring an answer in this case from the neural/fascial therapist's perspective is what or where is the matter with Geoffrey Watson? The matter being referred to is a matter of the physics of pain and illness.

Matter is substance. Physics texts describe it as that unchanging quantity of mass that has dimensions of weight, length, width, depth, and density. In pain, injury, and illness, any person can have several problems with matter. They are:

1. Too much matter
2. Not enough matter
3. Matter in wrong places
4. Poor quality of matter

As you may recognize, Geoffrey Watson was the victim of matter problem two (2) and matter problem four (4). Taking the four problems with physiological/pathological matter in order:

1. <u>Too much matter problems</u> can result from injuries causing compressions of the involved tissues. Such compressions compact the matter—the tissue substance. Tumors, warts, neoplasms, cysts, and polyps represent the laying down of too much matter. The accumulation of toxins from such items as the heavy minerals of iron, lead, and mercury, or emissions from bacteria, viruses, and fungi can and do bring on an increase in matter. Trauma to a body part can result in too much matter because the healing response may cause scar tissue to form where additional matter

cannot be tolerated.

2. The problem of not enough matter can result from congenital or genetic troubles. Also, the wearing down of matter by friction is a common difficulty encountered as in a scraped knee or a friction rub of toes in footgear. Injury can cause the tearing or removal of matter; Geoffrey Watson had tissue damaged and then it was removed as a result of his vehicular accident and the subsequent surgical operations he had undergone.

3. Matter in the wrong places may come on from the growth of cancerous tissue, atherosclerotic plaque that lines the walls of one's arteries, the deposition of fat on thighs or the abdomen, scarring from injury or operation, or some other form of illness and trauma.

4. Poor quality matter can result from poor food intake or general lack of nutrition. In the body, most of the time tissues do grow and replace themselves, but genetic defects, toxins, and other troubles can cause a lack of tissue or inadequate quality to the tissue. It's likely that Geoffrey Watson, from insufficient repair of tissues which had been traumatized, possessed such poor quality matter in his left shoulder and arm. As indicated, he became a victim of the physics of pain and illness.

Variables in Energy

All items in the universe have electromagnetic properties. Moreover, all living things produce energy. They need it to create for themselves warmth, mobility, growth, and the maintenance or replacement of tissues. However, problems with energy arise, too. There can be four particular difficulties:

1. A lack of energy
2. An excess of energy
3. Losses or breaks in energy
4. Blockage of energy

In the order of our listing, we shall explain the sources of these problems and, later on, how they may bring on pain and illness:

1. A lack of energy may come from the poor access to or insufficient intake of raw materials from nutrient sources. There may be an incomplete conversion of energy sources to energy itself. Perhaps there is some structural (matter) defect that involves the uptake, manufacture, or transport of energy.

2. An excess of energy may be due to blockage, causing energy not to be disbursed as it should. High energy may result from optimal fuel or good nutrition sources, too. High energy might arise from exercise or some other advantageous practices which ordinarily build health. Excessively high energy could bring on restimulation of emotions or actions such as anger, fear, joy or the use of stimulant drugs like caffeine, cocaine, and other harmful items.

3. Losses or breaks in energy can occur from illness or injuries. Injuries, for instance, are likely to break or damage nerves so as to disallow the normal energy pulse to flow along established channels. Further energy breaks may cause a pain and, in turn, the pain encourages repeated

spasms of muscles with a resultant further energy loss.

4. Blockage of energy from poor energy transport can build to an excess. Overabundant energy often gets lodged in a single tissue to stimulate associated symptoms. Energy blocks may be responsible for the lack of energy production, as well. Such insufficient energy production occurring from blockage may be typified by the ingestion of drugs and toxic agents. Most pharmaceutical agents have physiological blocking mechanisms. For example, beta-blockers, calcium channel blockers, tranquilizers, and other pharmaceuticals clearly impede or stop energy production and transmission. Additionally, toxins provide physical and physiological blocking activities of energy production and transmission. Drugs in sufficient doses may behave like toxins themselves.

Space and Time

In the universe there is connection not only with matter and energy but also with space and time. And these concepts relate to pain and illness, too.

What is space? While possessing a variety of definitions relating to astronomy, communications, printing, telegraphy, music, mathematics, and other human activities, the common understanding of space, says Webster's New Twentieth Century Dictionary, is that "it is the distance, interval, or area between or within things; the boundless expanse in which all objects exist and move; a portion of this, an area or volume for some particular purpose."

Well, space plays an important role in health and wellness, for too little space leads to loss of motion and loss of body fluid circulation. Both of these circumstances result in the loss of function. Too much space in the body would lead to instability, as well, and so beget weakness.

What is time? The same dictionary declares time to be "All the years of the past, present, and future; the passing of these taken as whole." In remaining healthy, time has a significant bearing on one's status. Illnesses and injuries, if not resolved, tend to become more entrenched so that they may move more matter over time. You might say that the body is like a book: when you do something good or bad for the body, it writes down what you have done (see illustration #3).

The best method for healing the body using time is to learn or recall the earliest event of the illness or injury and work to correct these initial factors. Such correction is like restoring a classic 1930 automobile that was in an accident in 1931. For restoration to the way it came from the showroom, you must go back to before the auto crash. Our claim is that you may bring about healing for yourself in the same way. The neural/fascial therapist helps you to recall your forgotten traumas by asking questions about big and small scars and other marks on the skin's surface or those thought scars lodged in your mind.

Misunderstood Thought

The mind harbors your thoughts, and you become

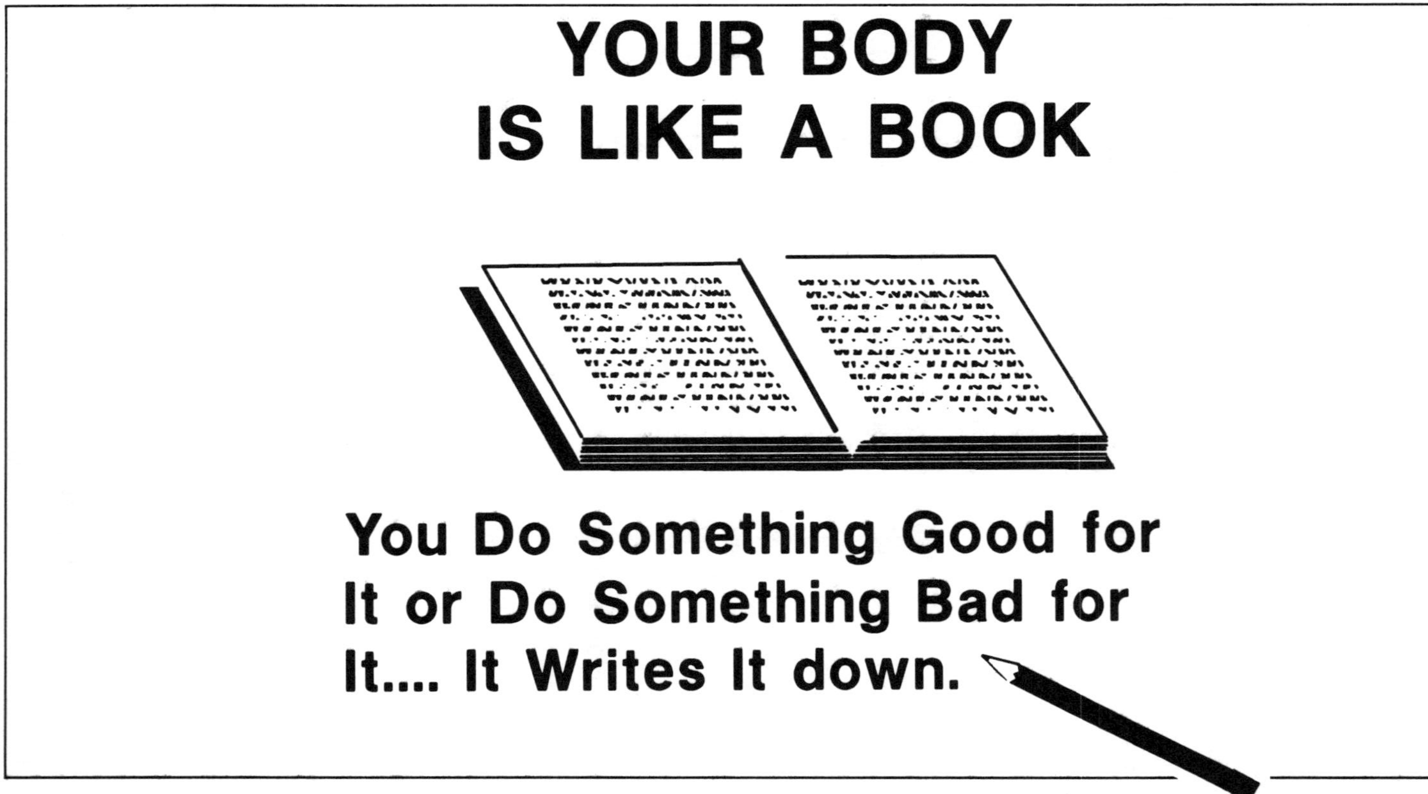
YOUR BODY
IS LIKE A BOOK
You Do Something Good for
It or Do Something Bad for
It.... It Writes It down.

Illustration #3 — Your body records all your physical and mental experiences.

your thoughts. Thought monitors, measures, directs, evaluates, plans, compares, records and files data on all the other physical factors as well as on the thought itself. Thought, like matter, energy, space, and time has limitless quantities of variation. Thought starts, stops, or continues all purposeful actions.

Of all the elements of the universe, thought is probably the most difficult to understand. It is most easily grasped as a concept if you consider that one's mind is like a video recorder. All the sights, sounds, emotions, smells, and touches to which you're exposed become recorded in the mind as if in a motion picture.

Through thought you may realize, for instance, that on certain occasions of deep feeling, high emotion, or from trauma in accidents, time seems to stop for an instant. The thought or emotion is recorded in your mind along with the matter, energy, space, and time alterations which happen with injuries, illnesses, or other significant events. The thought in an injury or an illness is an element of equal importance to any of the other physical elements of the universe.

The mind becomes a storehouse of psychosomatic arrangements. Numerous volumes have been written which are based on various psychosomatic illnesses. Some successful religions such as The First Church of Christ Scientists have a thought causation theory of illness and health. (See more of our thoughts on thought a little further along in this chapter.)

Correction of Matter, Energy, Space, Time and Thought Problems Which Cause Pain, Illness, and Disability

Inasmuch as everything in the universe relates to matter, energy, space, time, and thought, you should become aware that pain, illness, disability, and general dysfunction potentially take place when any of these universal elements become unbalanced. Straying from their normal operating state creates pathology. The goal of the mind-body-spirit correction is to restore all of these elements into balance—the return to homeostasis—with a minimum of disruption to the body.

Newton's First Law of Physics states that for every action there is a reaction. This is the reason that in biological medical practice a precise, gentle, corrective action is desired. Too much force from the health care practitioner possibly would further damage the patient's body and/or mind.

To correct matter in the universe or in the patient, you must first evaluate what is the matter with the matter. A therapist accomplishes this task by considering the other elements of energy, space, time and thought so as to create a mental picture of what happened before the first sign of pain or dysfunction began. Think how the mechanism of injury or illness would affect the body. For example, an injury that comes from being struck would produce a flattening of the structure (see illustration #4 & illustration #5). Thus, the best treatment for a striking injury would be for the therapist to use a hypodermic syringe and needle con-

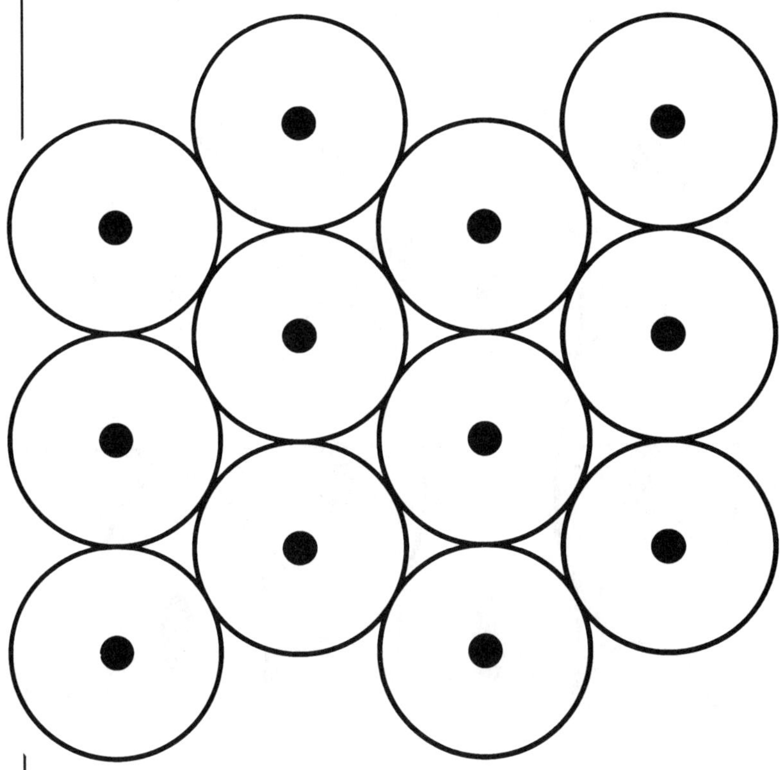

Illustration #4 — Graphic representing normal cell structure.

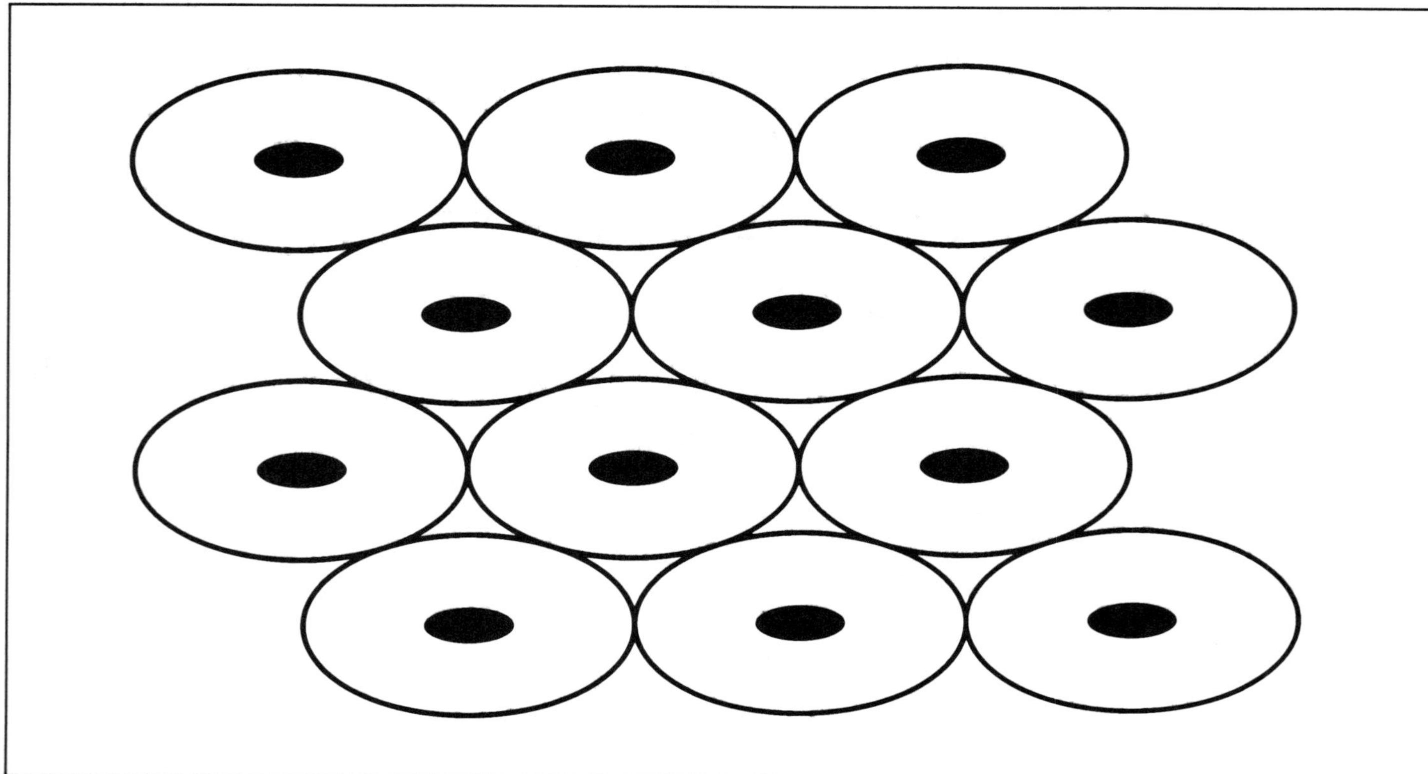

Illustration #5 — Graphic representing compressed cells from injury. Alteration of structure can cause altered function.

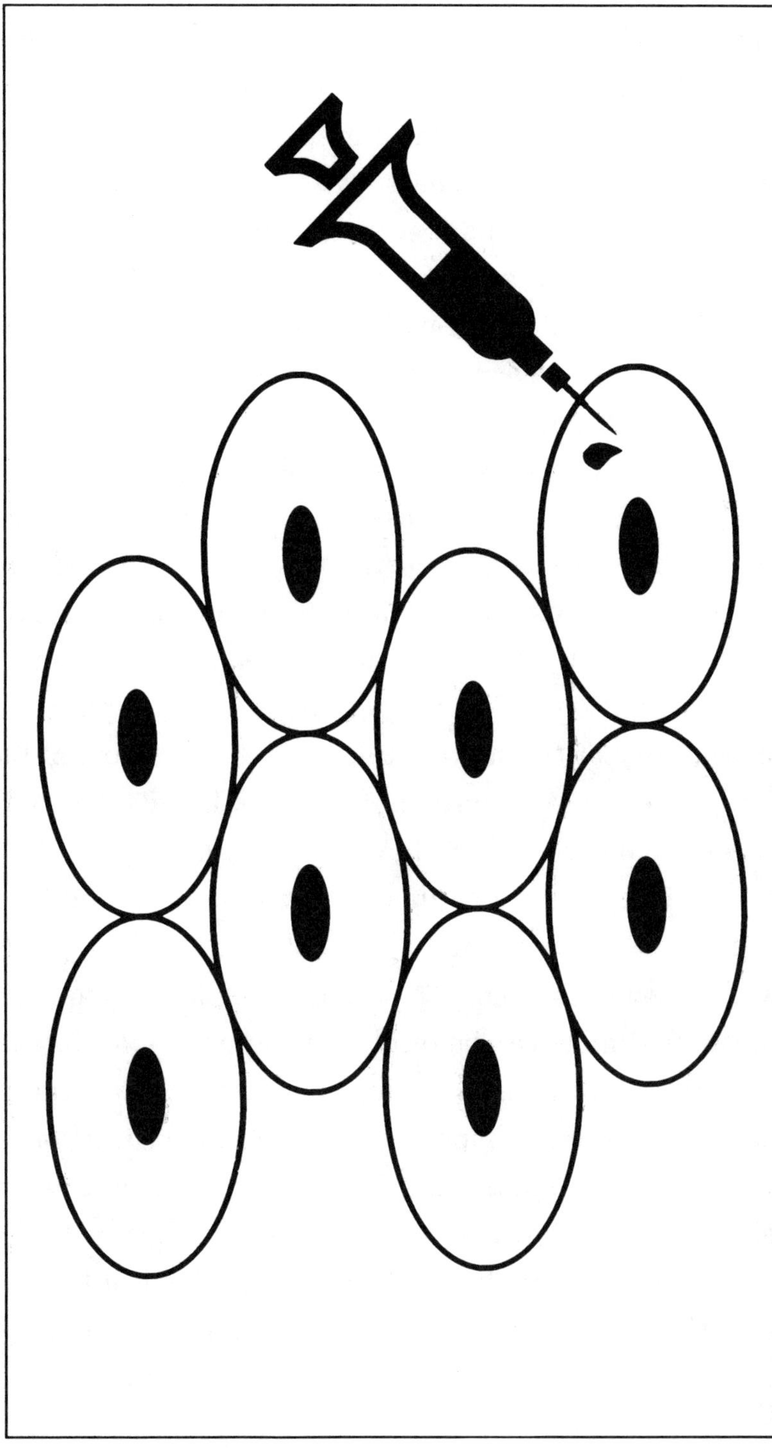

Illustration #6 — The hypodermic is an ideal tool to restore struction and function to compressed cells.

taining a solution for injection to restore the normal structure of the tissue (see illustration #6).

Lack of matter in the patient may be approached by optimizing nutrition. The body should be able to regrow required tissues as when reconstructive therapy is applied. Reconstructive therapy is a proven technique of stimulating the body to heal itself by placing tiny injections of irritants into the precise areas where matter is needed. Such irritation causes increased blood flow to the area; the blood releases growth factors which cause new tissues to build.

Excess matter could be approached by surgical removal or by other methods to increase blood flow and lymph flow so as to drain the accumulations of matter (toxins). Adding the element of space disburses and moves matter. Such an addition makes matter less dense; therefore, more permeability of the matter takes place by means of blood circulation and oxygenation. Wastes in less dense areas of matter are more easily removed.

Energy can be applied to living matter in different fashions so as to condense or disburse it. The work of Swedish scientist Bjorn Nordenstrum, M.D. shows that cancerous tumors can be resolved by applying low intensity electrical fields to them. Adding heat energy from an outside source such as from hyperthermia treatment units or from immunostimulation therapy have resolved tumors, as well. Using different forms of chemical energy has reduced or resolved tumors. Such chemical intervention would include chemotherapy, detoxification, intravenous chelation therapy, and nutritional approaches to remove matter. Substances such as dimethylsulfoxide (DMSO) can dissolve living calcifications and make them less dense.

Repeated physical or mental stress has been shown independently by the late medical scientists Drs. Wolfe and Selye to bring about calcification in the tissues. Toxic waste chemcials are known to accumulate in the human body and stimulate the growth of tumors (excess matter). The sun's energy is both light-giving and pathology-stimulating, since too much of it can cause matter accumulation in the form of skin cancer.

Then, time has cumulative effects, too, since it can force a change of living matter into one of degeneration. Time, as with other elements of the universe, may be advantageous or detrimental to the human condition, depending on its situation with the other physical elements. Gravity is not understood by most people to be a force, but the force of gravity over time has produced physical degenerations of the musculoskeletal system for many. Arthritics are illustrative of that truism.

Small corrective forces over time can produce significant results. Consider the workings of small amounts of water, for instance, and how they can keep living organisms alive and functioning. With no water present for a period of time, dehydration and death eventually must occur. Friction applied over time leads to calcification, loss of motion, and eventual fusion of joints and tissue. Because of another physical law of nature designated as "Wolfe's law," calcium in the body is moved to areas of stress. The stress may come from gravity, mechanical pressure, chemical alterations, or mental and emotional difficulties. Magnified over time, loss of function and pain must follow the continued pressure and tension of such stressors.

Inasmuch as everyone acknowledges that thought permeates all things related to mankind, it has been stated that "first there was the word, and the word was made MAN." As an interpretation of this phrasing: first there was thought (by the creator) and this thought was made into mankind. Some say that there are no accidents; everything happening in the universe happens for a reason. The assorted reasons represent thought or a lack of it.

Thought is the control which monitors, directs or misdirects destiny. Some physical scientists, even including metaphyscians, believe that thought is stored as chemicals in the brain; even proven by thoughts being altered by molecular changes in the chemical structures when electro-shock therapy is given to destroy memory.

The Hypodermic, a Precision Tool for Physical Imbalance Correction

Medical scientists have available a versatile tool for the correction of the physical elements. The hypodermic syringe and needle offer pin-point accuracy of application. Using reconstructive therapy, for instance, the hypodermic instrument handles matter by the stimulation of growth factors in precise areas of the tendons, ligaments, and joints, as detailed by the two of us in our best selling book, Pain, Pain Go Away.[2] Reconstructive therapy is shown to increase structure by up to 40 percent above normal, which may bring about improvement in clinical patients of over 100 percent increase in their structure and strength.

We assert that reconstructive therapy, administered by hypodermic, is the most effective, most beneficial, lowest-cost treatment for the loss of structure (tissue matter) in an extremely wide range of musculoskeletal problems. When all other therapies fail (including surgery, drugs, and manipulation) the hypodermic can and does deliver life-restoring energy to the cells.

The same occurrence takes place in neural/fascial therapy about which we are educating the reader here. For achieving instant pain relief, we advocate the use of strategically-placed local anesthetics by means of the hypodermic instrument. The reference book, the Physicians' Desk Reference, states that the mechanism of action of lidocaine, procaine, and other such local anesthetics by "stabilizing the neuronal membrane" restores action and energy to the body.[3] Thus, precise placement of stabilizing local anesthetics in and around nerves, blood vessels, tissues, and cells has a paramount reparative and energizing effect on the human organism. Patients receiving accurate, precise, neural therapeutic injections with lidocaine, procaine, and other local anesthetics frequently feel more alive with an increased sense of well being. They frequently describe the feeling of renewal as that of a weight or pressure being lifted off them.

Physician and scholar Franz Hopfer, M.D., D.D.S., of Vienna, Austria, who has written more scientific papers on neural/fascial therapy (in Germany, called "neural therapy") than anyone else in the world, states that neural therapy offers the body the greater amount of space that it requires. Since the hypodermic injects volumes of fluid which is largely incompressible, the injection procedure is an ideal way to cause more space to be created in tissue adversely affected by scars, injuries, compressive blows, calcifications, falls, and other trauma.

"Anesthetics eat torque," confirms the experienced neural/fascial therapist, James Carlson, D.O., of Knoxville, Tennessee, when advocating his application of injections. Dr. Carlson, indeed, has complained that the bio-electrical energy-adding powers of local anesthetics actually release pulling forces in the body perhaps allowing it to become too relaxed if excess anesthetic is used.

Linking Time and Thought by Means of the Hypodermic

Probably the best diagnostic tool utilized by the neural/fascial therapist is time. From taking the patient's medical history, the doctor learns of events that preceded the pain or loss of function. Painful trauma, infection, strong emotions, and other events that take place during anyone's time on earth are factors overcome by the therapist. Applying safe, near-painless injections as tests or questions asked of the body, he or she injects and observes what happens.

Frequently found is that there are a number of injuries or other defects upon which the hypodermic solution has dramatic, permanent, and instant pain-relieving results. Linking time and thought together with the hypodermic treatment, therefore, become one of the most significant tools for both diagnosis and treatment.

Thoughts as Sources of Pain and Dysfunction

Any health professional is aware that some destructive thoughts held by their patients can cause pain and dysfunction for the individual. Medical people attribute as much as 80 percent of all illness to psychosomatics (illness causes from the mind). Important psychological factors are connected to neural/fascial therapy. Precision of application of this treatment may be compared to the hunter who carefully practices for the hunt, tracks his quary's trail, camouflages himself in waiting, and finds success in the kill. Another hunter might simply go to the forest and shoot off his gun rapidly in a 360-degree circle, repeating to himself, "Gee, I hope something meaty runs into that ammunition."

In administering and/or writing of neural/fascial therapy, the co-authors have discovered that the mind component of illness underlies all pain and dysfunction for human beings. Numerous times in giving neural/fascial therapy, Dr. William Faber has experienced that his patient breaks into tears from remembering the details of emotions gone through at the time of injury, even though that event took place decades earlier. Dr. Faber also noticed that the correction of some imbalances relating to matter, energy, space, and time causes the patient to remember some other painful injury or event. Working to reveal the underlying difficulty sustained by the patient tends to penetrate deeply into problems as if one trouble masks from view other deeper problems which only surface after the initial disability is reduced or corrected. It's like peeling away the layers of an onion with the deeper dysfunctional layers being entirely different from others (see illustration #7).

We've used the video cassette recording as a metaphor for a person's collection of thoughts of pain and emotion. They exist on the reel of the individual's mind and if recorded over, pain and emotion become erased and healed. The best erasure occurs when the patient desires and seeks to change, looking for resolutions for his or her body and mind problems. Primarily this change takes place when the will is engaged, when the patient makes a picture of the event using the physical elements of matter, energy, space, time, and thought.

Intensification of that traumatic thought happens best when the patient thinks of all the physical elements which were present when injury occurred. Combined with neural/fascial therapy, such rethinking allows for the instant pain relief so desirable for anyone. Years more of pain and disability are relieved by the educated and skilled therapist's discriminating use of the hypodermic syringe and needle containing the appropriate local anesthetic. The most costly treatment for anyone seeking to be healed is from some particular therapy which does not work. We are pleased to report in all sincerity that neural/fascial therapy does work most of the time.

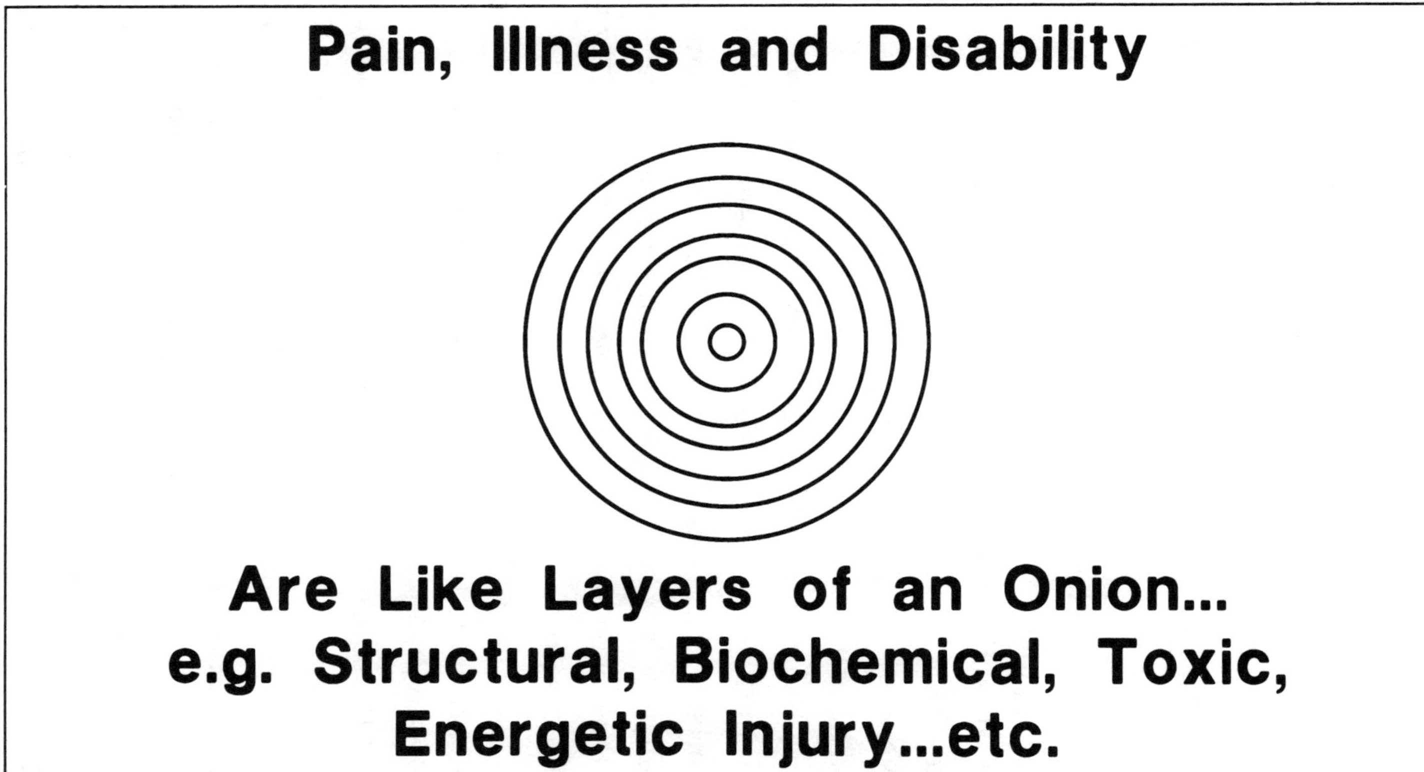

Illustration #7 — Often pain, illness and disability have multiple dimensions.

Chapter Two

FOLLOWING THE HEALING PATH

Are you following the path to greater health, wealth, and happiness? As we travel life's learning ways, undoubtedly, it is difficult to decide which is the best direction to take. This short chapter offers some concepts which may serve as an overall guide to help you on your way to sustained good health.

Before discussing the healing path, however, we present the patient case history of fifty-one-year-old Donald Alberts who lives in Davenport, Iowa. He is our current example of how healing concepts can work for anyone, even for those who are dubious or negative about following the healing path.

Dr. Jarka Odvarko, a well-known competent chiroprator from Bettendorf, Iowa, referred Donald Alberts to co-author William J. Faber, D.O. for a third medical opinion about the man's health problem. Mr. Alberts was needful of an alternative means of correcting his frustrating difficulty.

Because of vocal cord fatigue or some other reason that prior to then had remained undetermined, the patient's voice would just give out after he spoke for only 20 minutes. He had been a top salesman for a large clothing manufacturer, earning commissions of hundreds of thousands of dollars per year. With his voice fatigue ever present, however, Alberts' sales ability had dropped considerably. He ran out of voice stamina and seldom had enough vocalizing left to close the sale. The salesman's financial future was in big trouble; he knew it, and the manufacturer he represented was beginning to suspect as much.

Of course, Alberts went for medical consultation to what he considered was the best health care facility in midwestern America—possibly the most famous medical clinic in the world. The attending surgeon there told Alberts to undergo a vocal cord operation which would require him to remain silent for a minimum of six weeks. Clearly such a surgery was not what the salesman wanted to do. He was devastated in realizing that he would not be able to service his clothing accounts for this extended period. Competition was just itching to see him let down his guard, he knew, and he had already lost a few accounts by not being able to speak in any sustained fashion.

So, he sought a second medical opinion at a large university hospital. The throat surgeon at that place provided excellent service by filming the entire laryngoscopic examination. He showed Alberts how his vocal cords did not approximate well after he spoke for awhile. Feeling confident in the surgeon's abilities and this doctor's obvious humanism, the patient became enthusiastic about the outcome of treatment. He decided to undergo the surgery.

On the next visit for a final consultation, the university surgeon explained how he was going to make an incision across Alberts' throat so that the vocal cords could be openly manipulated to repair their defects. The patient accepted that he would need his throat cut. To ensure the best final result, however, it was necessary for Alberts to maintain six weeks of silence, he was told. Hearing that, Donald Alberts felt his heart drop down to his stomach. Despite his believing that here was the help that he needed and wanted, the same solution entailing financial jeopardy for his commission business was being offered. Consequently, Alberts decided that he could not accept the surgery at this time.

Jarka Odvarko, D.C., who was a family friend and had aided Alberts with some back problems, suggested that the patient's solution lay not with surgery but rather with medical attention that might successfully be administered by William J. Faber, D.O. It turns out that at the Milwaukee Pain Clinic, procedures really were much different. There, innovative biological medicine reigned.

The patient told his story while Dr. Faber listened attentively. This man's filled-in medical history sheets of information were then persued by the doctor. All new patients to the Milwaukee Pain Clinic are required to provide a full disclosure of their health problems, past and present. Among other health factors, Dr. Faber noted that Alberts had undergone a prior bowel obstruction surgery eight years before, an event that had left a considerable scar formation across his lower breast and upper abdomenal area.

Upon being asked, the patient removed his clothing to give access to the operative scars. The osteopathic physician rubbed Alberts' chest briskly along the scars which ran somewhat over the breast bone. The patient did not care for such rubbing in any way. It was uncomfortable. The scars were thick, had color in them, and were marked by many cross-hatch lines. The doctor then did muscle testing (kinesiology) on the scars while the patient touched them, showing clearly that he was weaker when he touched the scars, as opposed to when he did not.

Dr. Faber explained that the scars created both electrical short circuits and structural pulling as demonstrated by the clinical examinations and tests. He showed how the structural pulling of the scars of the abdomen could alone be the cause of the patient's voice fatigue. "It's like having a weight tied to your shirt all the time," Dr. Faber said (see illustratin #8).

He added, "Neural/fascial therapy may be just the thing to correct this condition being created by the scars." Then he explained that the injections served a dual purpose. They structurally loosened the scars and the lidocaine solution to be injected simultaneously repaired the electrical short circuits. The injections, said Dr. Faber, were both diagnositic and therapeutic.

Not to be swayed from the course of potential treatment that he still had in his mind, Alberts asked if the injections would interfere with his proposed throat surgery. Dr. Faber replied, "Absolutely not. You can have your surgery any time you want."

The patient agreed to receiving a series of injections with local anesthesia and returned one week later for more. They had caused him no difficulty whatsoever. In fact, he stated, his voice was stronger and and lasted longer. In

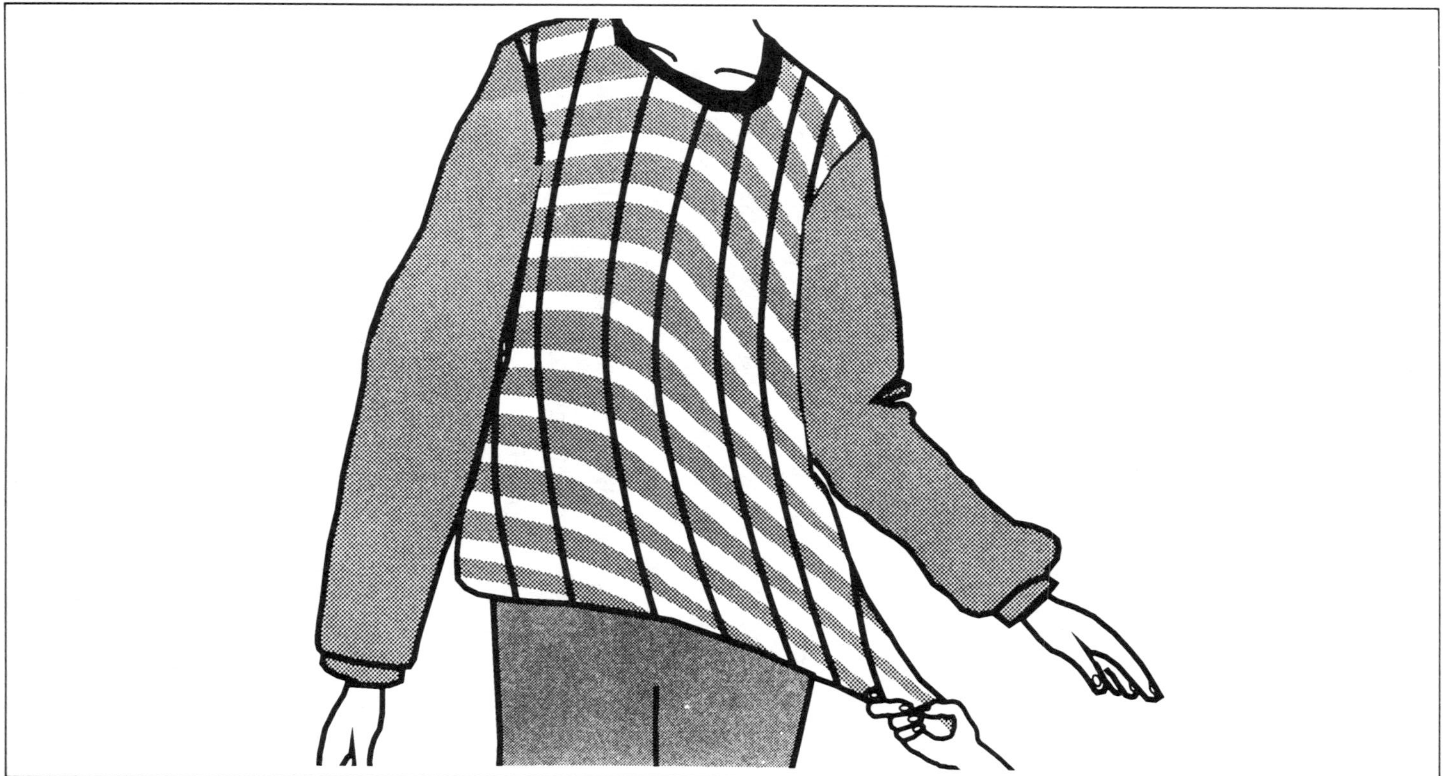

Illustration #8 — A scar or an injury can distort the entire structure and cause pain and disability remote from the causative area.

timing himself, he could speak for an hour without feeling vocal cord fatigue. Three more treatments resolved the problem altogether for him.

Within the month Donald Alberts gave a speech to his Kiwanis Club and spoke nonstop for several hours afterward in greeting his friends and fellow members whom he had not seen for a long time. Mr. Alberts decided against undergoing the throat surgery. He declared that he just did not need it anymore.

Everything that Happens to You Counts

In Chapter One we said that your body is like a book: You do something good for it or do something bad for it.... It writes it down. A permanent record is filed in your brain and in various parts of your body where trauma has taken place (see illustration #3). Whether you notice it or not, everything counts—nothing that happens to you loses significance. That is why it's so important to build healthfulness on a steady basis rather than wait for the inevitable sickness or injury that comes to all of us at some time during the course of living. Once you become ill, you'll be forced to seek crisis care. Why wait for a crisis to take care of your health?

Besides, the health insurance policy you carry, for which you've probably been paying high premiums or for which you've accepted less of a salary because of the policy being a company fringe benefit, most likely is going to be dictating the type of medical care you can receive. As far as the health insurance industry is concerned, there is no freedom of choice of how its clients may be treated. Your health insurance carrier usually dictates who may give you treatment and what kind of care you're going to receive. Sure, surgery may be compensated for, but it's not often that innovative medical procedures such as preventive health maintenance or nutritional therapy is paid out or reimbursed. It's likely that insurance coverage you own should not be named "health insurance care" but rather "sickness crisis care" (see illustration #9).

An injury or illness that you sustain has many aspects to it. As we explained in the first chapter, the pain, illness, and disability which may become part of your life's experience are like the layers of an onion. They become lodged deeply in your psyche and make themselves an integral part of your body's wisdom. There are all types of trauma wisdom: structural, biochemical, toxic, energetic, injury, and more (see illustration #7).

What Did Donald Alberts Learn?

All the aspects of an illness or injury must be corrected in order to receive a full measure of healing. This is the lesson learned by Dr. Faber's patient, Donald Alberts. Having a voice that failed had brought Mr. Alberts to two high-powered surgeons who were ready to give him empirical treatment—surgery to the local area of disturbance. That's how they were trained and what they knew to perform—to do some slicing on the vocal cords.

If he had consulted an allopathic internist who used

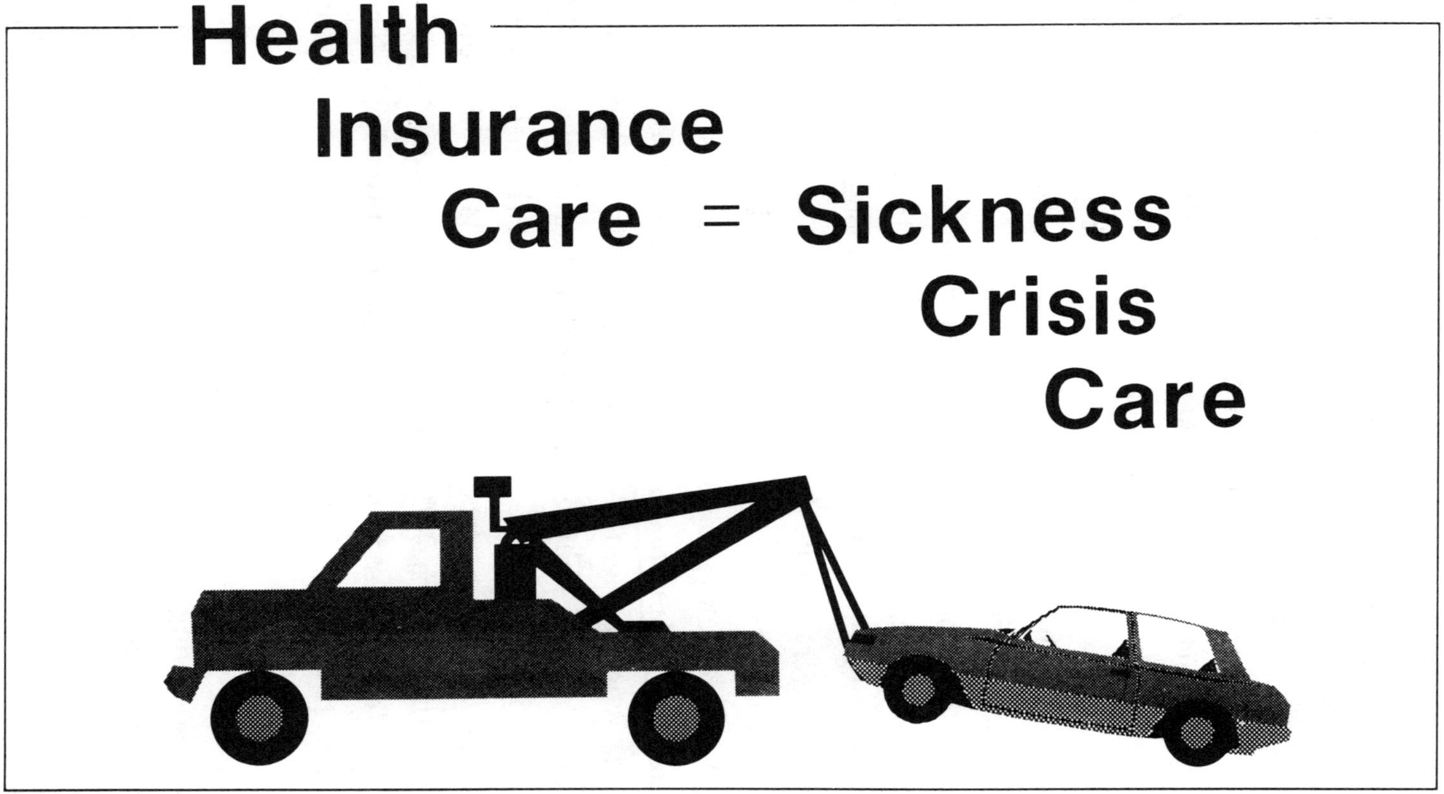

Illustration #9 — Health insurance is designed not to provide health but rather care during sickness and injury.

drug therapy rather than surgery, the patient would have been offered pharmaceutical products as the treatment regimen. Taking drugs, what would have happened to the patient then? Drugs are synthetic forms of toximolecular agents which tend to block processes within the body's healing cycle. Any drug itself is never completely cleared from the body and this leads to further problems. It's another trauma—a sort of poisoning—with which your body and mind must cope.

You should realize that when the only instrument a doctor or another type of health care technician has to work with is a hammer, then any patient who comes along looks to that specialist like a nail.

At the Milwaukee Pain Clinic, Dr. Faber gives preference to unraveling the patients' health problems with non-toxic biological methods. John L. Sessions, D.O. of Kirbyville, Texas, whose patient, Geoffrey Watson, we described in that important first chapter on the physics of medicine, was trained in exactly the same way. All of the osteopathic doctors or medical doctors educated in the use of neural/fascial therapy are skilled in this manner, as well. You will meet a few of them in forthcoming pages of this book. The patient cases that they've provided are intriguing to read and identify with.

As with the onion analogy that we used earlier, when the underlying layers of a person's health problem are exposed various symptoms come to the fore. They show themselves and are made ready to get solved. With help from the therapist, your body does the solving. One by one the problems go away and their symptoms disappear forever by use of neural/fascial therapy.

You know, of course, that you can't feel your headache at that moment when a brick drops on your foot (see illustration #10). So, why do you feel the symptom that brings you to a doctor for treatment? Because when an illness or an injury persists it's often the "straw that breaks the camel's back" in action. Your body just can't take abuse anymore and it lets you know how it feels by producing discomfort, dysfunction, or another set of signs and symptoms of some kind.

The Pain Threshold and Your State of Being "OK"

Thus, one may have no pain after injury until the individual's "pain threshold is met." It's practically a series of stair steps into injury and illness. You experience the initiator of trauma or sickness; then a multiplier of dysfunctional circumstances sets in; there is a third multiplier of the trauma; plus another eventially takes hold which may consist of body abuse which could include smoking cigarettes, drinking alcohol, using recreational drugs, being malnourished from eating mostly junk food, death of a much-loved spouse, or experiencing some other life-change crisis. So the intensity of traumatic body abuse increases until you reach the threshold at which your body declares: "I'm mad as hell, and I'm not going to take it anymore!" So, you experience pain (see illustration #11).

Here is an explanation of the pain threshold stated

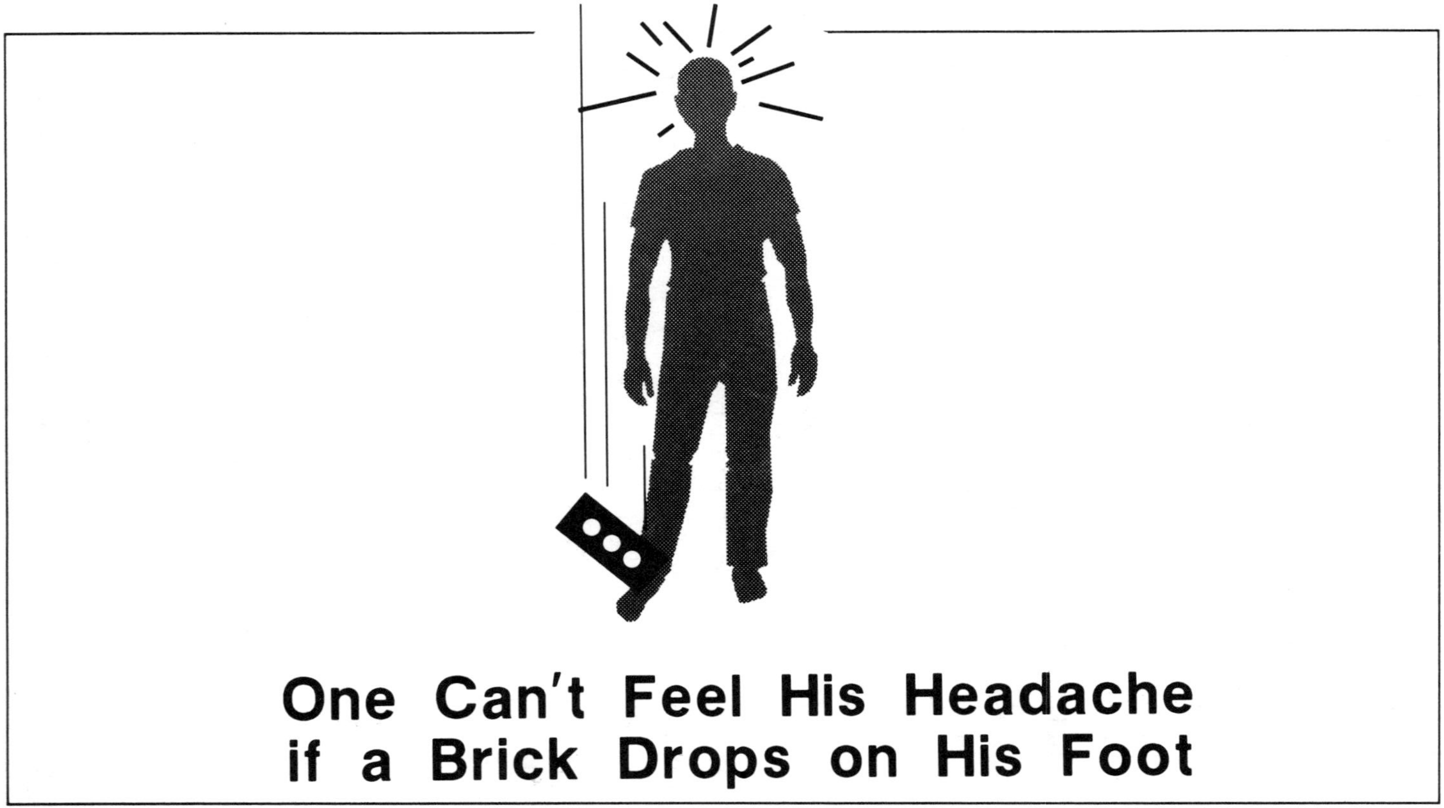

Illustration #10 — Frequently the pain and symptoms change during the course of biological neural/fascial therapy treatments.

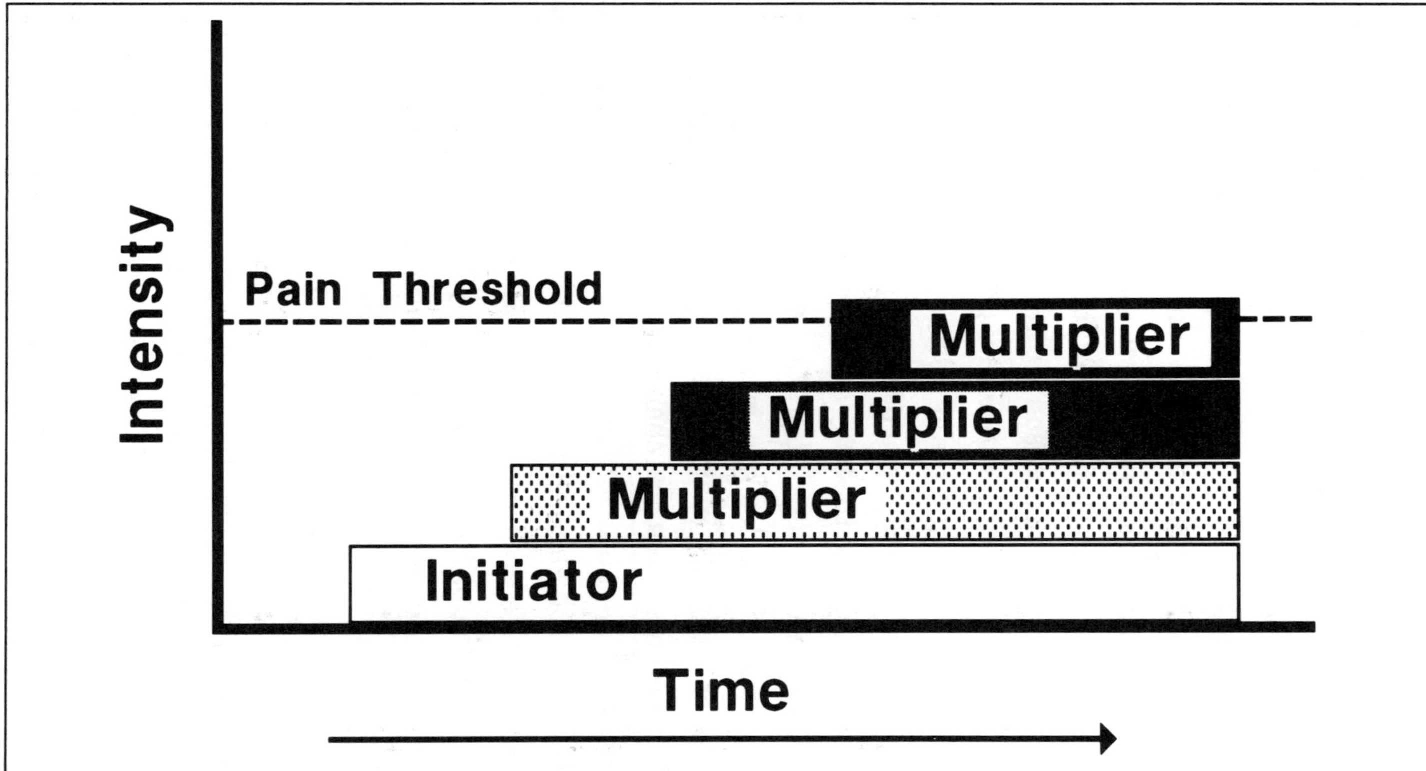

Illustration #11 — Often chronic pain is produced by a series of injuries or problems over time.

another way: illness and pain are like the tip of an iceberg. When they appear they have been in the making for a long time (see illustration #12).

From the first chapter we know that molecules occupy space. There are good molecules and bad. The good ones are natural substances which have existed on the earth for thousands of years (maybe millions), and many of them become a part of your personal physiology. Your body has a use for them either in its structure or as fuel. Food molecules like bricks for a house build a strong body, and you remain in a state of "OKness" when the toxic load of bad molecules is contained within the body's storage areas. No overt symptoms are noticed (see illustration #13).

Bad molecules are waste products from the body, drugs of all kinds, man-made substances that pollute the environment, unnatural chemicals, and certain toxic components found in nature. The body has a number of methods to detoxify and eliminate these bad molecules. When more bad molecules are in the body than can be eliminated, the baddies pile up. For a time you may continue with no overt symptoms because the body has found space in which to hold these bad molecules. Eventually, of course, you run out of space and the baddies spill over in the form of disease symptoms.

You require ongoing detoxification through the usual elimination processes of your physiology. If effective elimination is not achieved, the bad body molecules continue to pile up until, indeed, the body really does run out of storage space. Illness, pain, and dysfunction follow simply because

CHRONIC PAIN AND ILLNESS ARE LIKE AN ICEBERG

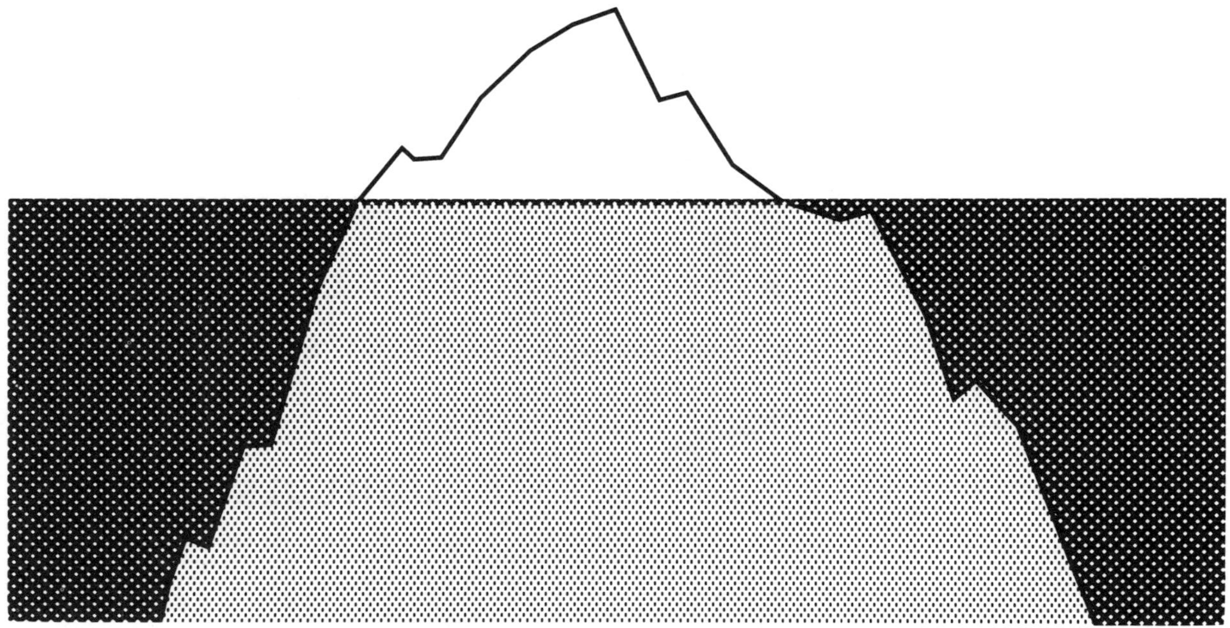

Illustration #12 — Pain and disability reveal themselves only when their magnitude is great enough that compensation is no longer possible.

Illustration

A state of "OKness" is present when toxic load is contained within the body's storage areas. No overt symptoms are noticed.

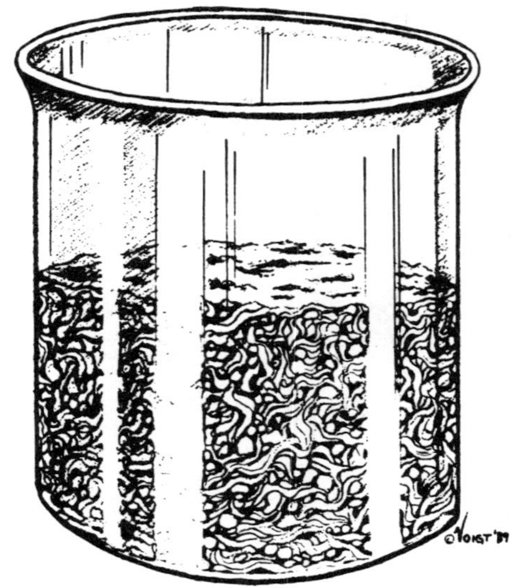

Illustration #13 — The body has the ability to contain amounts of toxins without symptoms.

the toxic load capacity is exceeded with resulting signs and symptoms of disease (see illustration #14).

The research undertaken by biological practitioners shows that a clean body has no toxins in its storage areas. The body and mind have optimal healing ability and a reserve resistance to illness (see illustration #15).

How to Tell You Are Receiving the Right Treatment

John Diamond, M.D., of Pleasantville, New York has told us that the body does not lie, and he is telling the truth.[1] Careful observation of your body's actions, reactions, feelings, functions, and complaints will enable you to reveal answers to questions such as "Am I giving myself a quality of life that's beneficial?" "What must I do to increase my chances of dying in a state of youthfulness but at a very old age?" "How can I tell if I'm going through the right treatment?" These are fair questions to ask your body, and the method for acquiring their answers has been explained to medical science by Franz Hopfer, M.D., D.D.S., of Vienna, Austria.

This Austrian physician/dentist has developed a method of determination by using neural therapy, a modification of which we have adapted as well. Then, we have taken his method some steps further and renamed the advancement "neural/fascial therapy". Using normalization injection treatment of nerves, tissues, and organs, we find specific corrective mechanisms which offer clear answers to what the body wants by providing immediate results. Either

Illustration #

Toxic load capacity is exceeded with resulting symptoms and illness present.

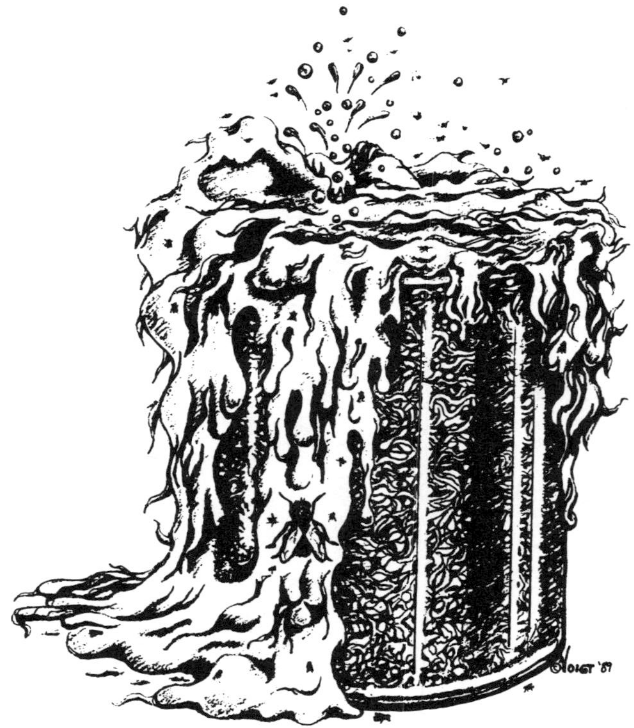

Illustration #14 — It is often only when the bodies toxic capacity is exceeded that symptoms and disability appear.

Illustration #

A clean body has no toxins and optimal healing ability.

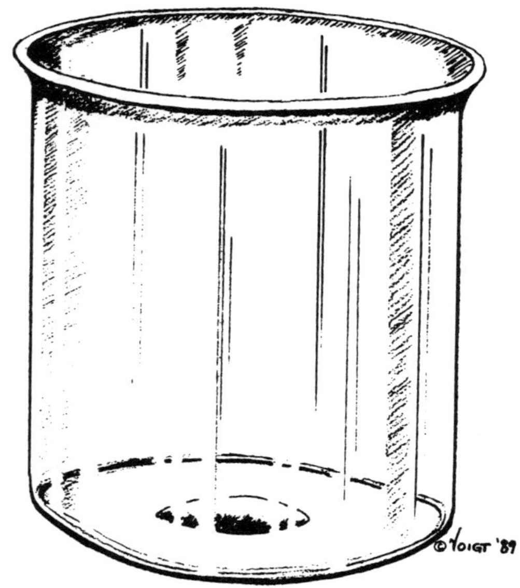

Illustration #15 — A clean body is obtained by using detoxification methods and leads to optimal health.

you experience instant pain relief or you don't. Immediate relief is the body's "YES" answer to the question: "How can I tell if I'm going through the right treatment?"

Looking at the beginning or the base line level of pain and dysfunction, the treatment required is applied to the source of trouble. It may be an injury or a scar of some kind. From the administered treatment—any type—there will be an initial reaction that could aggravate the condition temporarily and cause a worsening of symptoms. Or, suddenly you may feel and see an improvement of signs and symptoms—experience them disappearing altogether.

The key as to whether you are going to have success is how your body is behaving in about a week's time. If your body feels less pain and improves in function after approximately one week above the baseline of the illustration, this probably is the body's "YES" answer (see illustration #16). Often the time period required for an accurate answer is seven days because the body needs this period to utilize and/or adjust to the injected solution that's administered during neural/fascial therapy. A shorter time interval may be used by more experienced doctors.

The treatment may be given to you by the doctor until the maximal result is obtained. How does the therapist know when to stop? The body says it has had enough with a "NO" response (see illustration #17). If symptoms and dysfunction return to the starting baseline or below, no further aid can be obtained by repeating the treatment at this time. The body has stated, "I need and want something else as treatment."

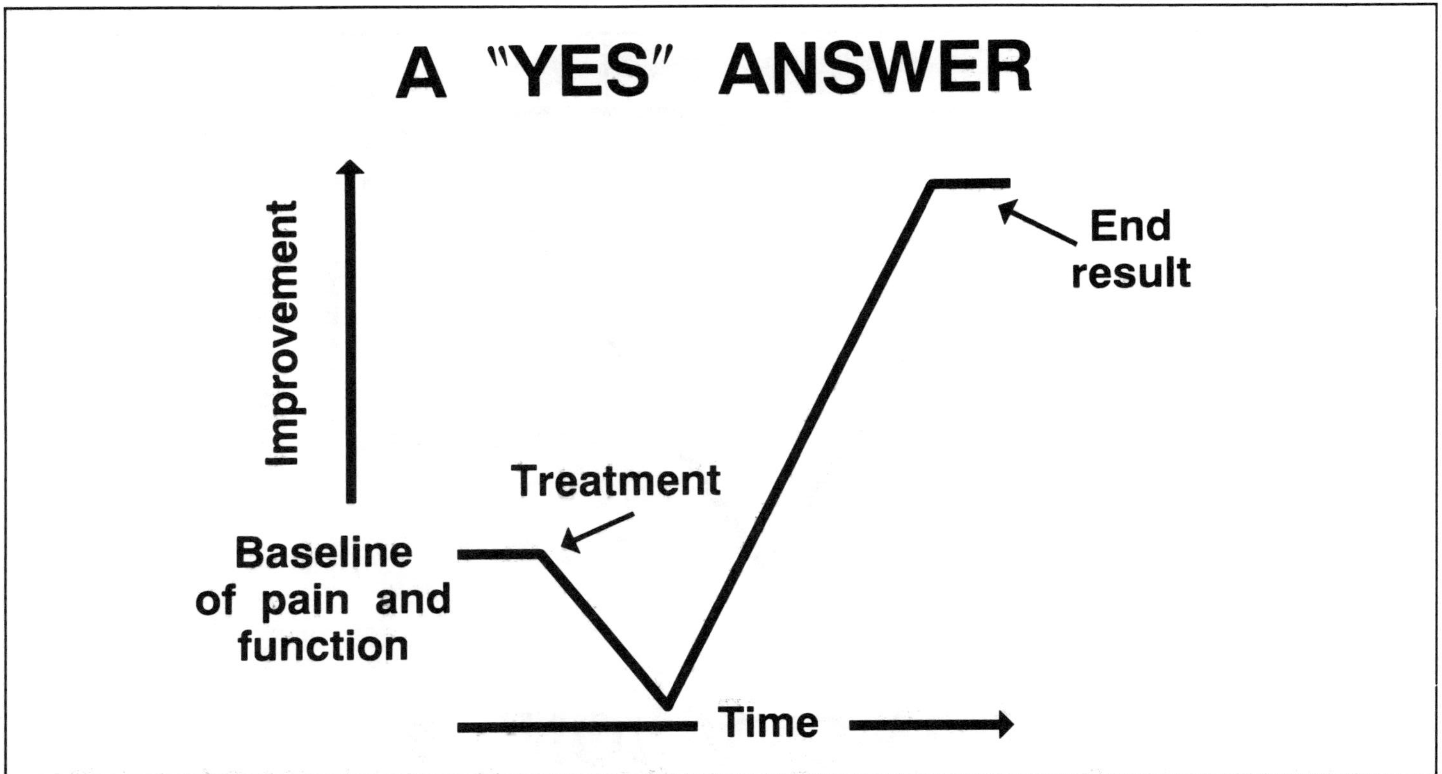

Illustration #16 — The body responds with a "yes" when improvement persists after the treatment has ended.

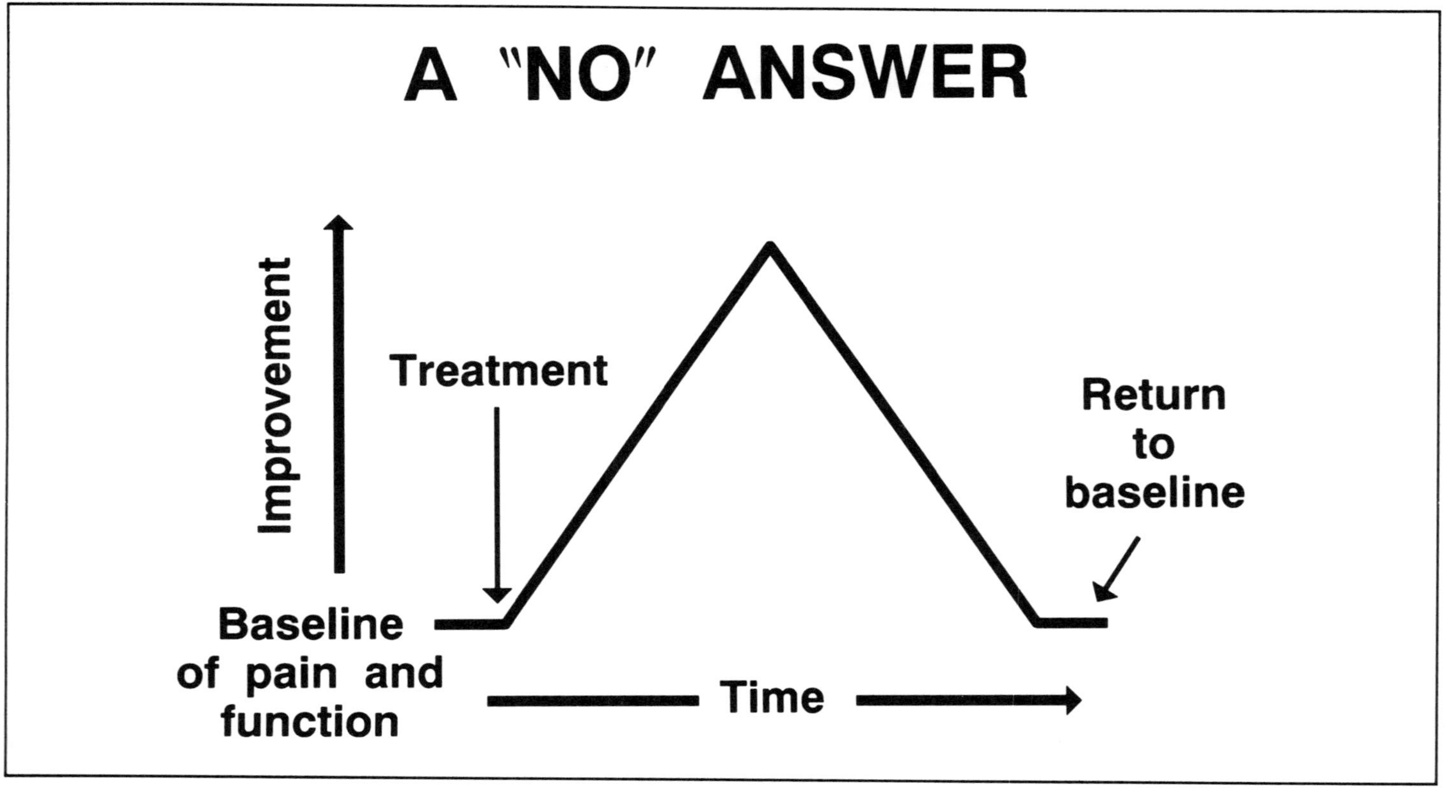

Illustration #17 — The body responds with a "no" when no improvement results after a treatment has ended.

There is a third response the body may offer, too. It is, "I don't know!" This means the body is so toxic and sick that it can't really give a "YES" or "NO" answer. In this case the doctor will find it necessary to lower the total toxic load of his patient's body and build up the individual's defensive immune system. Such a situation may occur even in young people because the altered environment experienced by our industrialized society has become so ridden with pollutants, atherogens, allergens, carcinogens, and other causes of degenerative diseases. Sometimes a "flare" may occur which is a worsening in some area. This indicates other problems which must be corrected.

The Physical Body in Ideal Balance

In the physical sense the human body in balance may be thought of as a perfect triangle (see illustration #18). It is held up and together by its physcial structure which is the foundation upon which all internal systems function. Defects in structure will result in defective function.

What makes viable structure? Biochemistry of quality. Inasmuch as it's known that we are what we eat and absorb, the body's structure is constantly being built up and torn down by the quality of what we ingest. Biochemical processes assimilate the fuel provided by food and produce energy. Defects in biochemistry will cause faulty structure. The nervous system goes awry because the nerves and brain direct actions within this faulty biochemical structure.

It's like conditions at the control tower in an airport.

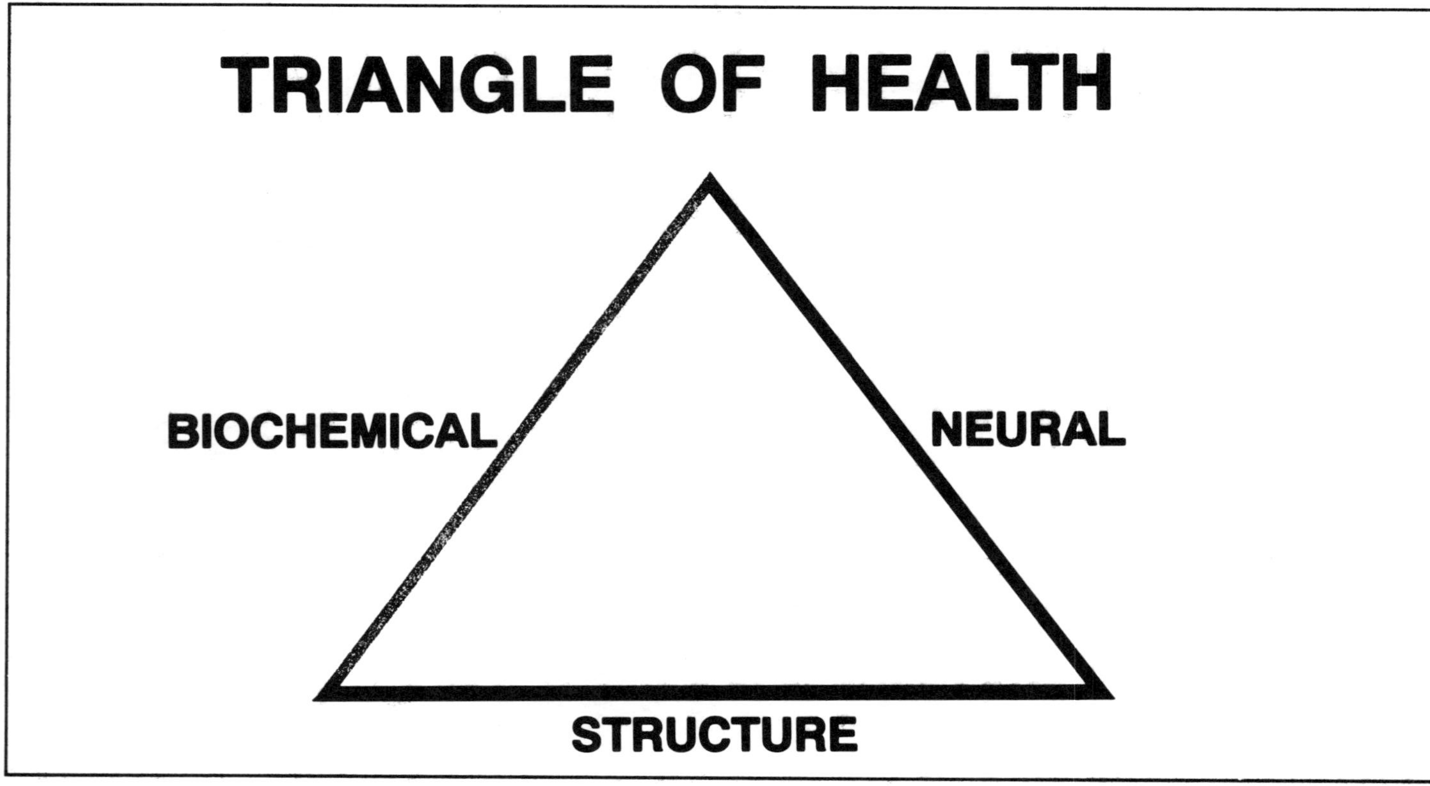

Illustration# 18 — Ideal physical health is represented by a balance of structure, biochemistry and neural systems. We stand on our structure which is fed, energized and replaced by our biochemistry. We are monitored and directed by our neural system.

The controllers (our nerves and brain) observe and direct the activities within the body and mind so that abnormal function is bound to develop when the systems involved with structure and biochemistry get out of their ideal balance. Incidentally, the mind and spirit are main contributors to appropriate balance and function.

Now, you may wonder about the sources of injury, chronic illness, various traumas, and scars; how far do they go back so as to still be a producer of discomforting symptoms and signs? As we shall see in Chapter Three, they can go back quite a long way, even to a point that one's conscious mind has totally forgotten their occurrence; but the subconsciousness has not.

Chapter Three

PAIN FROM REMOTE SOURCES

In his teaching text, Neural Focal Dentistry, the noted German-Hispanic physician and odontologist, Ernesto Adler, M.D., D.D.S., tells the story of a certain Dr. Badia of Barcelona, Spain who became renown for his unique diagnoses and therapies. Typical was the case of a 62-year-old, stooped-shouldered Spaniard named Carlos who sported a flowing black mustache, a gaunt face, bifocal eyeglasses, and a small pot belly. Carlos was suffering from malaise, serious gastrointestinal difficulties, and a general body weakness.

Accompanied by his brother, Carlos visited Dr. Badia and told of his personal gastrointestinal distress as he patted his protruding belly.

"Tell me your story again," said Dr. Badia.

Carlos did!

Dr. Badia listened and then replied, "Tell me your story again."

Somewhat impatient, Carlos repeated his tale.

Observing the patient, Dr. Badia said, "Tell me your story again."

Exhibiting great annoyance and by now in a deeply irritated mood, Carlos described his symptoms a fourth time.

Dr. Badia said, "Tell me your story once more."

Carlos would have none of that and lost his temper, shouting at the doctor, "I came here for you to heal me, and not for you to mimic or have fun with me."

Doctor Badia responded, "My friend, your gastric troubles will disappear if you shave off your mustache."

With that, Carlos uttered insults at the doctor and spat out vulgarities which would make any listener cower. He stormed out of Dr. Badia's office vowing to expose him as a charlatan.

Still, the patient's brother who had heard good reports about the doctor's cures before the current incident had occurred, gradually convinced Carlos to get rid of his proud mustache.

Amazingly, within days of the barbering, the patient found that all of his discomforts disappeared. He quickly gained strength, no longer felt unwell, and did not experience gastrointestinal distress in any way.

It wasn't a placebo effect, Doctor Badia explained later to Dr. Adler. It turns out that the patient, while speaking, often wetted his lips with his tongue, which simultaneously made contact with his mustache. Having an acute clinical eye, Dr. Badia had noticed that the middle-aged man's head hair and mustache were dyed with a chemical which he knew usually caused toxic symptoms if taken internally. Obviously it was the poisonous dye which entered the patient's body through his tongue that was causing his symptoms of internal difficulties.

Pain from Remote Sources

Dr. Badia's diagnosis and treatment demonstrate that health problems and their corrections can come from remote sources. You can find pain relief, for instance, by giving treatment to a part of the body distant from the area that hurts. To illustrate, in acquiring toothache relief, apply deep pressure to a point located between the thumb and index finger. This point is called "Ho-ku" by acupuncturists, who frequently use it to treat dental pain.

Bringing this concept of eliminating pain by treating remote sources of pathology to your present personal interest in instant pain relief, let us tell you the story of Waukesha, Wisconsin resident Sandy Moody, age 49, an assembly line worker in an automobile factory. Sandy visited the Milwaukee Pain Clinic and Metabolic Research Center in Milwaukee, Wisconsin to consult with medical director William J. Faber, D.O. Her complaint was a constant feeling of severe pain on the soles of both feet, especially her heels. The pain was particularly bad in the morning upon arising. For the previous six months it just hurt her so much that she sought help, in turn, from a podiatrist, a neurologist, and an orthopedist but with no good result coming from the three consultations. Medication that had been prescribed didn't do her any good. Sandy still felt bad pain in the heels, on the outside edge of the soles, and in the middle of the metatarsal heads of both feet.

Dr. Faber's examination of her feet proved negative for some physical disturbance except for a slight decrease in the extremities' range of motion. There was no point tenderness; rather, pain seemed to come from inside the tissues. Her circulation and standard nerve tests were normal. A careful history of Sandy's health throughout life was elicited and recorded on patient history forms. The forms' typical questions included: "Have you ever experienced foot and ankle problems before?" She had not! "What surgery and injuries have you had?" "What accidents and injuries did you go through?" "What illnesses, drugs used, or allergic reactions have occurred during your life?"

Getting answers to these questions, Dr. Faber asked Sandy about her digestion, bowel and urine elimination, and other pertinent factors relating to her physiology.

A search of the patient's body revealed a scar on her leg, which she recalled coming from an old dog bite when she was a teenager. Abdominal examination revealed a small scar from a laporoscopy examination (checking of the abdominal cavity by insertion of a lighted, hollow metal instrument). Careful examination of her scalp revealed a roughness of the frontal area in the hair line. It was a slightly different color from the rest of her skin.

Dr. Faber asked, "What is this roughness on your head?" At first Sandy responded, "Nothing!" She didn't remember any trauma, until his continued rubbing of her head at a cycle of eight hertz (the natural magnetic vibration of the earth) brought back her memory. "Twenty years ago," Sandy said, "I had a car accident and my head went through the windshield. I healed up OK and forgot the incident."

Rubbing some more, Dr. Faber declared, "This is what

I want to treat—the minor scar on your head. I find no intrinsic problem with your feet. Your foot trouble most likely comes from your scalp."

The rubbing caused Sandy Moody to speak up some more with the admonition, "You know, at times I notice that I want my husband to rub my head. It gives comfort to my feet."

To Dr. Faber, having come in contact with such circumstances a few hundred times before, Mrs. Moody's statement did not sound peculiar at all.

The dog bite and laporoscopy scars also were suspected as complicating factors — known as "interference fields"—to be discussed in Chapter Two — but Sandy's nearly invisible head scar, because it felt sensitive to touch, was very suspect of causing her foot trouble.

The patient showed some evidence of having various systemic disorders of allergy, liver dysfunction (dark circles under the eyes), and poor digestion. Still, Sandy did live a relatively wholesome lifestyle in that she drank distilled water, avoided sodapop and coffee, ate mostly unprocessed foods, exercised regularly, and had fairly regular bowel habits. Dr. Faber offered Sandy Moody the new/old German neural/fascial repair therapy (also to be described in the second chapter) to achieve instant removal of her lower limb pain.

Treatment was administered to the mashed-type, nearly invisible scar in her hair line, and the corrective procedure immediately produced a pain-free effect. The patient was able to walk without any foot discomfort. Sandy bounced around the office as if skipping rope and was bursting with joy at her recovery. Laughing happily, she said, "I can't believe it; my feet and heels don't have aching or hurt at all."

Four more neural/fascial treatments given a week apart totally and permanently resolved the patient's lower limb problem. And Dr. Faber never even treated her feet.

Chapter Four

NEW/OLD GERMAN NEURAL/FASCIAL THERAPY

While dressing to attend church one Sunday morning, 50-year-old Mona Manley, a rancher's wife residing on the Big Island of Hawaii, experienced an abrupt onset of severely disabling pain in her left flank, an area between the pelvis and the ribs, that doubled her over. This region above the left buttock had not been injured at all, and Mrs. Manley could not recall ever feeling such an uncomfortable symptom before. The pain stayed with her even as she visited a family practice physician located near to her ranch.

Believing that the pain problem was kidney-related, the doctor initially diagnosed Mrs. Manley as suffering from renal colic. She was treated with the appropriate analgesics and encouraged to increase her fluid intake. Inspite of these measures, however, the pain continued unrelentingly throughout the week. The local physician therefore referred his patient to a urologist, William Yarbrough, M.D. of Honolulu, across the interisland waterway, on the Island of Oahu, Hawaii.

Dr. Yarbrough completed a full physical examination, including clinical and laboratory workups. He could find no cause for Mona Manley's severe left flank pain, which by now was radiating up and down the buttock. Believing it not to be a urological involvement but rather gynecologically-connected, Dr. Yarbrough referred Mrs. Manley to gynecologist/obstetrician Joseph A. Brock, M.D. of Honolulu, a Fellow of the American College of Gynecology and Obstetrics.

As it happens, Dr. Brock, who also is a Fellow of the American Academy of Neurological and Orthopaedic Surgeons, had just completed a preceptorship in neural/fascial therapy at Dr. William J. Faber's pain clinic in Milwaukee. Describing what transpired with Mona Manley, Dr. Brock writes: "I did a thorough gynecological examination and found nothing amiss in this regard with the patient. Instead, I did notice that she had several well-healed scars at places where surgeries had been performed. Her past medical history included six normal pregnancies and vaginal deliveries from 1956 through 1961, a hysterectomy in 1964, a cholecystectomy (gall bladder removal) in 1970, a lumbar discectomy (disc removal) in 1974, another lumbar discectomy in 1977, a foot surgery in 1980, and a cervical discectomy in 1983. The scars were not painful and had never bothered her. There were no tender swellings beneath them.

"I suspected that this patient might be harboring a neural interference field in one of the scars, and so I briefly explained the concept of our new/old German neural/fascial therapy to her and her spouse. At this point they were both open to just about anything since the pain had really worn her down," Dr. Brock said.

"I elected to inject the vertical scar over her spine from the previous discectomies and her well-healed cholecystectomy scar (in the right upper quadrant of her abdomen) using the appropriate dilution of local anesthetic (preservative free)," explained Dr. Brock. "In 30 seconds, she had complete remission of the left flank pain. The patient and her husband were taken aback with amazement at the speed and permanency of this treatment. I advised them to remain in Honolulu overnight for follow up. The next day, however, there was no recurrence of pain and no more treatment was needed."

"I saw Mona Manley again three months later, and she was still pain free. Checking with her recently, she has remained without any return of the pain in her left buttock and flank," Dr. Brock advised us.

What Is Neural/Fascial Therapy?

The procedure that Dr. Brock used, Neural/fascial therapy, involves the manipulation of nerves and tissue employing a small gauge needle for administering tiny amounts of diluted local anesthetic. This administration is not for purposes of temporarily numbing nerve sensitivities but rather for a greater physiological purpose which first requires some explanation in order to fully answer the question: What is neural/fascial therapy?

Every science textbook teaches students that all cells including the cellular components of nerves, blood vessels, bones, muscles, and connective tissues have a bioelectric gradient. This gradient in each cell consists of the electronegative charges of ions which we mentioned in the Introduction. Such ions are provided by negative atomic particles from minerals coating the cell's outside membrane and electropositive charges from minerals along the membrane's inside. Thus, a cell is like a battery with potential energy between the positive and negative charges separated by its membrane wall (see illustration #19).

When some disruption of the cellular wall or membrane which separates the negative and positive charged particles occurs and a hole or opening develops, the normal bioelectrical potential reverses. Negative charges now rush through the opening into the cell and positive charges rush out. In a microsecond an alarm signal is propagated to the spinal cord and brain saying, "Start functioning!" "Turn on!" Or more often, "Short circuit and give pain!" With the latter response, such a short circuiting or miscommunication in the body's electrical system gives rise to more permanent pathology and the onset of chronic pain (see illustration #20).

This recurrent situation for their patients was observed by two German medical scholars, Ferdinand Huneke, M.D. and Walter Huneke, M.D. In 1925, the Huneke brothers experimented on their sister who suffered with chronic migraine headaches. They injected a small amount of procaine (invented in 1906) into her vein, which instantly resolved her migraine permanently.[1] Before this event, medical scientists erroneously believed that intravenously administered procaine and other local anesthetics were harmful. The two Drs. Huneke defined neural/fascial therapy using procaine as a means of correcting disruptions of

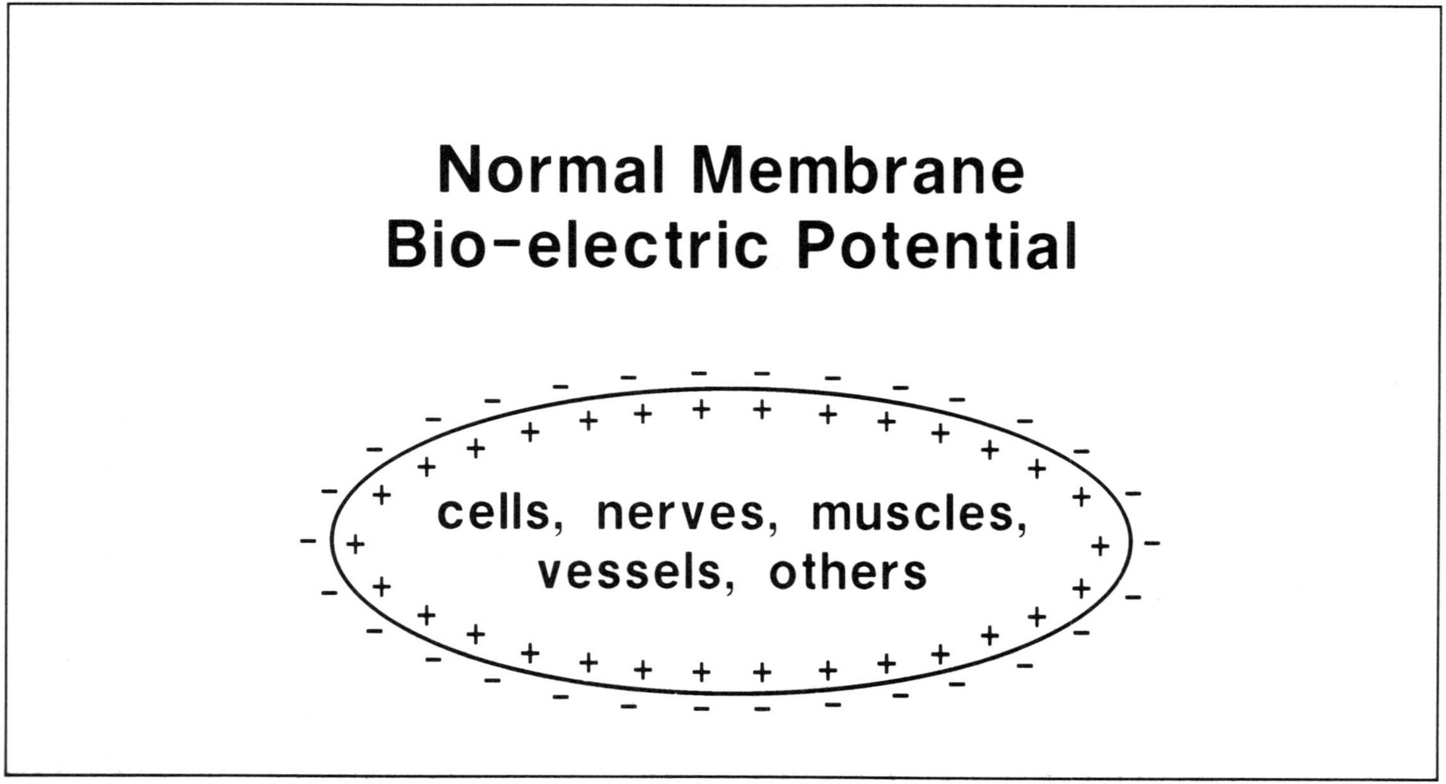

Illustration #19 — All living cells and tissues maintain a biochemical potential charge.

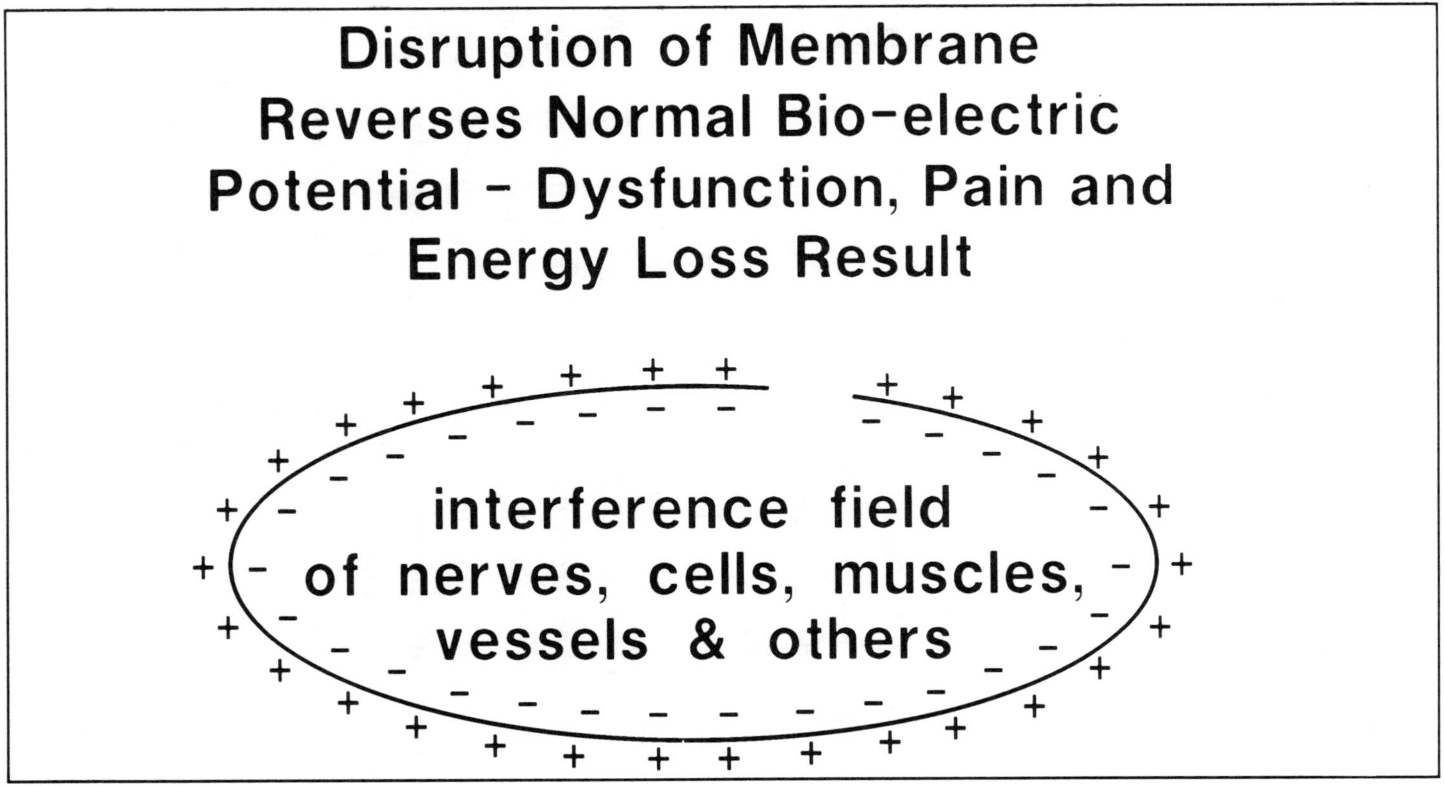

Illustration #20 — Disruption of the cell membrane causes the cell to turn on signaling pain messages to the brain.

normal bioelectric balance of the cellular nerve membranes or energy flow. Such disruptions or breaks in the electrical field, they stated, may be caused by surgical operations (cutting cell walls), injuries, infections, fractures, toxins, sunburns, and scars. All of these defects produce interference fields (breaks in the electrical energy flow), producing short circuits in the nervous system and fascial tissue.

Summarizing Neural/Fascial Therapy to this Point

In summary, therefore, neural/fascial therapy is the injection of local anesthetics similar to those employed by dentists to desensitize teeth. The anesthetic injections are applied to carefully selected points of the body, by means of which it is often possible to cure or greatly ameliorate a large variety of predominantly chronic conditions.

Since about 1928 when the Huneke brothers first described their treatment in the publication, Medizinische Welt (Medical World), under the title, "Unexpected Remote Therapeutic Effects of Local Anesthesia," there have been extensive research programs and numerous other publications about this new medical science. However, nearly all the research and writing has been performed in Germany (with some relatively small amount done in other European countries and a little in South America). The result is that German-speaking physicians make up the majority of exponents for neural/fascial therapy. It is hardly known in North America.

As we have explained, the injection material is a local

anesthetic consisting of either procaine, lidocaine, XylocaineTM, or one of the other agents utilized by dentistry to cause a numbing of the teeth and gums. These local anesthetics, while obviously used in the United States for their deadening effect, also possess the ability to bring about changes in the function of individual nerves of the autonomic nervous system and consequently in the cells and tissues served by the particular body system.

A large amount of medical literature documents these physiological changes brought on by injection of the family of solutions whose name ends with the suffix "caine". The caine solution changes occur at the cellular level by means of the repolarization of depolarized cell membranes, a highly complicated natural phenomenon. The inherent complexity and functional organization of the neural/fascial regulatory system is used by the administering doctor during the clinical application of this treatment to his patient.

How Neural/Fascial Therapy Is Given

Injections, which themselves cause no discomfort, are given into segments of the body harboring areas of pain. The injections of local anesthetic are made directly into a site of pain such as that affecting tendon, muscle, and ligament or into the skin or in the neighborhood of the afferent nerves or into and around the autonomic plexuses or sympathetic chains of the nerves. The doctor's aim in giving such an injection is to reach the patient's autonomic network at whatever point a presumed functional block exists in it.

An illustration of this functional block penetration occurred in the clinical jaw-locking case of Margareutte Wilshire, a 36-year-old married school teacher residing in Knoxville, Tennessee. She is the daughter of a prominent Nashville, Tennessee specialist in internal medicine and in the decade gone by had presented him with two grandchildren, the light of his life.

In the spring of 1990 Mrs Wilshire visited a dentist for routine attention to her teeth. She lay back in the dental chair, opened her mouth at his request, heard a click at the intersection of her upper and lower jaw bones, and suddenly found that she could not close her mouth. This lockjaw position caused her acute pain. The dentist grew alarmed, attempted jawbone manipulation, tried to wedge her mouth closed, and finally became highly aggitated at his failure to do anything to ease the patient's discomfort. With sign language, grunts, and futile movements of her tongue, she did manage to advise that this situation had never happened to her before. Finally, the dentist hit on the idea that osteopathic treatment might unlock the patient's facial joints, and he strode to the telephone seeking assistance from James A. Carlson, D.O. of Knoxville, who is a pioneering practitioner often at the cutting edge of advances in biological medicine.

Dr. Carlson consented to aid the patient, if possible, and she walked through Knoxville's sunny streets with her mouth fastened in the wide open position. He discovered that Mrs. Wilshire's jaw was dislocated backward from its original axis.

Among questions Dr. Carlson asked and that Mrs. Wilshire wrote answers to were, "Do you have any scars that I don't see?" She advised him of a hysterectomy performed on her three years before. The woman thought it unusual but did give permission for the osteopathic physician to examine her belly scar. He saw a thick, dense scar running from the upper pubic line to the umbilicus. He said, "I know you may think it sounds crazy, but if you allow me to inject that scar we'll get your mouth to unlock real quick." She agreed!

Using a neural/fascial therapy technique, Dr. Carlson injected the patient's belly scar with lidocaine. When she sat up, immediately her jaw clicked again, the temporomandibular joint corrected itself, and Margareutte Wilshire found that she no longer had a lockjaw problem. She returned to the dentist for a resumption of her dental work.

Segmental treatment of the body in the region of the patient's scar had relieved tension of her myofascial pattern in the woman's face. Mrs. Wilshire's usual range of motion of the jaw joints were restored and the pain evaporated. This is standard procedure when neural/fascial therapists apply their techniques to individual segments of the body which are involved with interferring pathology.

Treating Body Segments

Skin injection (referred to by neural/fascial therapy's proponents as "quaddle" therapy because quaddles or tiny hives are raised on the skin surface) affects autonomic function. This happens by means of segmental reflex channels located in areas related to the body segment giving pain. When the doctor is successful with his technique, the patient experiences his or her pain disappear or there is a substantial amelioration of symptoms. Pain relief greatly outlasts the anesthetic effect. In fact, the freedom from pain often continues for days, weeks, months, or permanently.

For Margareutte Wilshire, the correction has stayed in place permanently. If symptoms had recurred, however, Dr. Carlson would have repeated his administration of the same injections. The effect of repeated injections becomes progressively more complete and will last for a longer period until pain never comes back.

As another example of the pain-relieving effect of care with neural/fascial therapy, be aware of backache as a positively responding condition to this procedure. Neural/Fascial therapy is practically specific for eliminating backaches of all types and locations. It's well-known that most adult spines show some arthritic changes, although the X-ray films of arthritic spines may or may not show calcareous deposits on the bones or around the intervertebral joints. When correctly-sited injections of a local anesthetic are given to a patient during the course of neural/fascial therapy for backache, the pain and related symptoms such as limitation of movement, will disappear or be greatly improved. Yet, the X-ray film findings taken long after the treatment is over do remain unchanged. The pain of backache may be gone forever, but the deposits of calcium probably remain. However, clinically Dr. Faber has noticed the resolution of crepitus has taken place. Often there is a marked decrease of the grinding sensation (crepitus) that frequently is noted in arthritic joints. That's because the injections have been given into interference fields created by the presence of one or more scars on or within the patients body. Body and head scars which set up fields of interference are among the subjects of our next chapter.

Chapter Five

INTERFERENCE FIELDS AND THE LIGHTNING REACTION

Arturo Sabattini of San Diego, California, a 44-year-old plumbing contractor, suffered acutely from a severe, immobilizing shoulder condition. "Artie" (as his wife and friends usually called him) could not use his right arm or shoulder in more than a 20-degree basis from his normal range of motion. His plumbing business was suffering because being right-handed, Artie had difficulty lifting and raising heavy objects, especially when he had to install overhead piping in a basement.

Mrs. Sabattini made an appointment for her husband to consult with William C. Kubitschek, D.O., of San Marcos, California. She had heard good reports about Dr. Kubitschek's use of a "different" kind of injection technique for just such trouble as being experienced by Artie.

Following his examination and evaluation of the patient, Dr. Kubitschek came to a judgment that Mr. Sabattini would, indeed, benefit from neural/fascial therapy. As a test, the man was given a minute priming dose of local anesthesia intravenously, with no signs of allergic response. Following this, the area of his pain about the subscapular glenohumoral area of the shoulder was injected. Additionally injected was a large area of scar tissue from a previous cyst removal near the bottom of the right scapula (shoulder blade).

It turns out that the scar of that oldtime cyst operation was just the right place to unblock the body flow of electrical nerve impulses for Artie Sabbatini. He experienced what neural/fascial therapiest call a "lightning reaction." Within three minutes Artie had total relief of his pain. Within ten minutes he was able to move his arm through the full range of motion, and he did it with absolutely no discomfort. The patient was amazed at how quickly this new/old German neural/fascial therapy had taken hold.

In fact, he was being exposed to the instant pain relief of what proponents of the treatment look for, the lightning reaction—rapid therapeutic response. "He has a brother who had severely acute shoulder pain all the time and who had learned to live with it," Dr. Kubitschek told us. But not Arturo Sabbatini; "lightning" had struck for him, and his shoulder pain never returned. Rapid therapeutic response had broken through the interference field which was blocking the plumber's usual nerve impulses.

Fields of Nerve Impulse Interference

The human being is a living organism who functions only through communication between his body parts. (Do you know the song lyrics: "The knee bone's connected to the foot bone"? These song words have truth to them.) Neural/fascial therapy affects this system of communication. The

Drs. Huneke concepts include the presence of interference fields related to pathologies that produce symptoms in a person suffering agonies of pain. Huneke has put forth that past injury to any group of cells can lead to present stress on and heightened vulnerability to irritation of other areas of the body. The site of past injury becomes the focus of the interference field and is most commonly encountered as visible scar tissue.

Scar tissue then becomes the site of injection. Thus, a childhood tonsillitis (and/or tonsillectomy) may in later life be the cause of a refractory polyarthritis, migraine headache, or asthma. In that case the presenting condition will respond inadequately or not at all to the usual allopathic therapies or physical therapy. In contrast, an injection of local anesthetic solution such as 1 percent or 2 percent procaine or 1 percent lidocaine—always without adrenalin—into the tonsillectomy scars or the tonsillar poles will give instant pain relief.

This instant relief is known as a lightning reaction—rapid therapeutic response—also referred to after its discoverers, as the "Huneke phenomenon."[1]

To be accepted as a lightning reaction, the effect of instant pain relief must last for at least 20 hours on the body and eight hours in the case of a dental interference field. If there is any recurrence of pain after this period, the Huneke rule for it to be a true lightning reaction is that the effect of a repetition of the previous injection procedure must exceed the first injection in duration and effectiveness. Pain relief must be complete and immediate.

A single treatment may be sufficient, or a series of repeat treatments of an interference field at lengthening intervals will lead to a cure of the condition, in so far as this still remains anatomically possible. Most scars do act as interferring agents and set up interference fields.

How to Tell if Scars Are Interference Fields

There are signs, tipoffs, or hallmarks that certain scars are acting as interferencial (interference) field agents. The following are interferencial field hallmarks:

(1) A usual scar's color changes from purple to red to light red to pink to pale to white. The interferencial scar's color may be other than pale white which persists in its off-color even after two years.

(2) A scar that adhers to tissue and fails to move like other more normal surrounding tissues will probably be producing an interferencial field.

(3) If there are hatch marks or tension lines in or around the scar you have another sign of a break in the electrical energy flow.

(4) Torque on the scar that is present shows it's likely producing an interferencial field.

(5) If the patient notices there is pain, numbness, tingling, or other strange feelings and alterations in sensorium in or around a scar there is interference with electrical energy flow.

(6) Any scar that tests positively to some bioelectric examination as with the Voll machine, the Vega ma-

chine, or the Dermatron electrical acupuncture device is behaving as an agent of interference.

(7) Physical examination as with applied kinesiology that shows positive responses points up scar interference. (Refer to Chapter Five for a full discussion of kinesiology.)

(8) Some therapies which tune into the body rhythms such as with cranial/sacral therapy may give a signal of interferencial scarring. (The doctor must watch for false positives which are actually negatives).

(9) Any fracture site, bone bruise, puncture, infection site, frostbite, tonsil removal, and dental extraction must be considered a scar capable of producing physiological short circuits.

(10) Any moles, pimples, acne scars, chickenpox scars, wrinkles, vacination scars, or other lesions that should not be there must be considered as building interference fields.

(11) Any totally asymptomatic scars are probably causing nerve energy interference.

(12) Such interference with nerve energy as it passes along neurons and through fascial planes must give rise to signs and symptoms of illness, especially pain, as a result of the blocking and accumulation of nerve impulses.

Signs and Symptoms of Nerve Energy Flow Interference

Discovering that you possess your share of interferencial scarring, you will be able to attribute a variety of discomforts , disabilities, and dysfunctions to them. For example, the following are signs and symptoms of nerve energy flow interference contributed by the many types of scars and imperfections already listed:

(1) Stiffness, pulling, soreness, numbness, tingling, cramping, or other sensations which slowly or immediately follow a health impairment such as injury, surgery, toxic exposure, sunburn, or other events,

(2) Dysfunction or loss of function of a part or organ after a health impairment event,

(3) An unexplained acute pain,

(4) Other types of health impairments, defects, or traumas.

To appreciate why these signs and symptoms of nerve energy flow interference occur, realize that a scar can act like a patch on a balloon. It can exert a pulling pressure which can cause a marked change in the entire shape and function of that balloon. Another way of seeing it is that the scar or patch controls the entire balloon. The balloon becomes a slave to that scar (see illustration #21). In the same way, sewing up a body suit as with stitching together the skin after a surgical operation causes that body suit to become tighter and tighter. Soon you lose your compensatory activities because you can't move in that stitched-together body suit.

So what do you think it's like for a person undergoing one operation after another? The individual has only so much body, right? After surgery, does the body get looser or tighter (see illustration #21)?

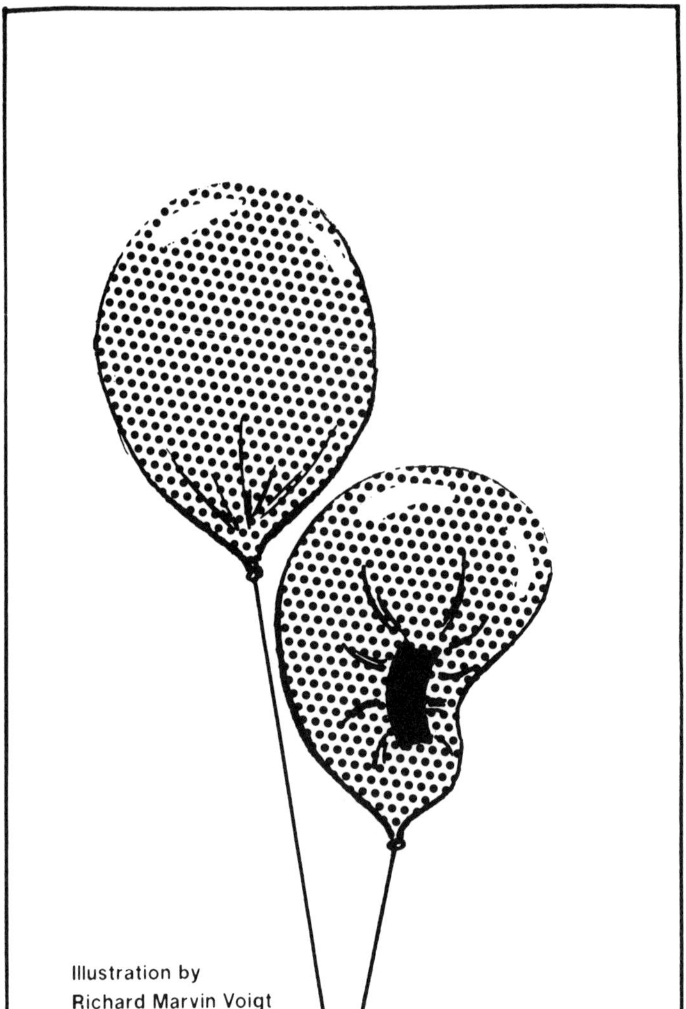

A scar can act like a patch on a balloon.
It can exert a pulling pressure which can
cause marked change in shape and function.

Illustration #21 — A scar can control the entire shape of a living structure.

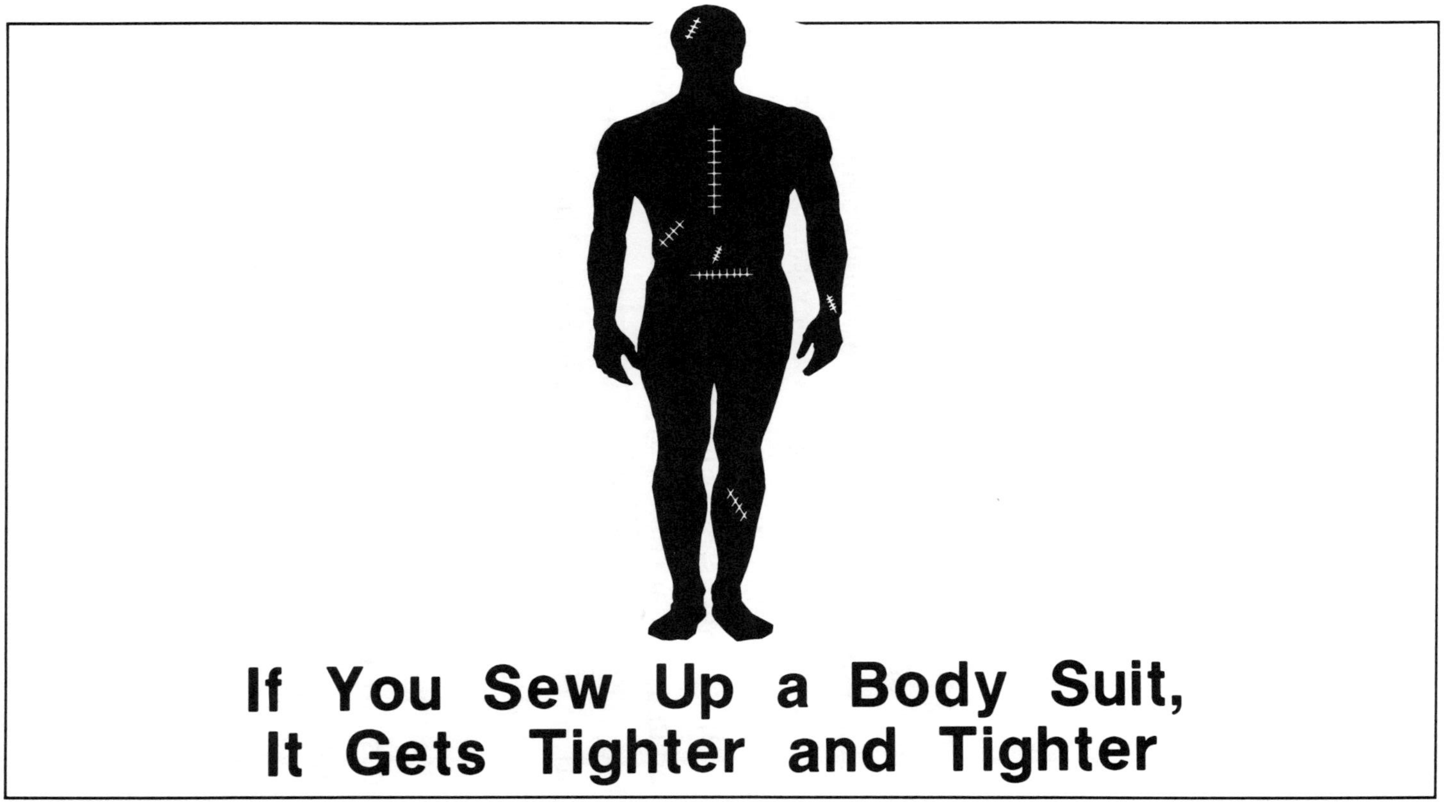

Illustration #22 — Multiple surgeries can lead to lack of space which puts tension on nerves and tissue causing pain and disability.

Interference Field Sources of Signs and Symptoms

There are common critical situations which predispose themselves to creating interference fields and the signs and symptoms that accompany such sources. They include the following:

(1) Abdominal scars that bring on gas, belching, hiatus hernia discomfort, chronic indigestion, postural pain, lack of endurance, and inflexibility of the body in general as typically manifested by a young woman's inability to dance the "boogy woogy" after hysterectomy or ovectomy. (Scarring pulls the woman's body too tightly.)

(2) Chest scars such as those occurring with the fashionable coronary artery bypass operation. (Tightness of the body shell or skin around the chest may mimic the sensations of angina pectoris or myocardial infarction.)

(3) Dental scars, Tonsil scars, adenoid scars, and head scars can create migraine, visual disturbances, jaw dysfunction, tics, paralysis, spasms, weakness, pain, personality changes, eye ptosis, head and neck structural malfunction, and tinnitus.

(4) Circulatory system organ scarring.

These sources of signs and symptoms in a tight body suit violate the rules of space. In the physical world, if something exists it must occupy space. Length, depth, width, and weight are all characteristics of matter. Matter therefore can accumulate and take up more space. If there is room for it, a body's actions and reactions are all right. If there is insufficient room, problems begin since situations relating to physiology simply get too tight inside the body shell, and overflow congestion conditions exist.

While what we've just said seems simple enough in real life, it's not so simple in the microscopic world. Microscopic organisms such as bacteria, viruses, fungi, parasites all take up space. If they accumulate to excess, they cannot be contained and lumps, tumors, cysts, blockages, and other abnormalities can result. When such excess growth of tissue occurs, a cardinal principle of osteopathic medicine comes into play.

"THE RULE OF THE ARTERY IS SUPREME."

This principle means that where there is good blood circulation and drainage, there is health and homeostasis. But poor blood circulation results in low oxygen, insufficient nutrients, inadequate drainage of waste products, and eventual pathological symptoms and signs such as pain, swelling, tumors, degeneration, and disease—even cancer.

Scars, burns, injuries, surgery, sprains, strains, infections, fractures, toxins, and other insults to the body that are subtle or overt can produce a too tight condition that pulls on nerves and chokes off the blood supply to cause dysfunction and pain. It really is a matter of space when pathology manifested by signs and symptoms is involved. Lack of space on the body's outer surface or internally brings on stress. In turn, stressors stimulate the formation of calcification which is the topic of Chapter Six that follows.

Chapter Six

THE STRESS OF LIFE

For over 20 years, Maria Foster of Madison, Wisconsin, a 52-year-old merchandise manager for that city's biggest department store, suffered from tinnitus, a ringing in her left ear, and an accompanying hearing loss. Mrs. Foster had undergone a surgery on the ear for cholesteatoma, a mass consisting mainly of cellular debris in which cholesterol crystals are present in the tumor. Her cholesteatoma had developed in the middle ear and, by pressure, it had caused destruction of surrounding structures.

The ear operation failed to produce any significant change for Mrs. Foster, and she lived with her problem until her brother reported that his own tinnitus was eliminated by treatment received at the Milwaukee Pain Clinic and Metabolic Research Center. Consequently, seeking the same sort of help, the woman consulted with William J. Faber, D.O.

Dr. Faber examined Mrs. Foster and questioned her to learn her full health history. She admitted to hitting her head many years previously. The doctor found a loss of motion in the area of the surgery and in the same place as the old injury. This finding was significant to him.

Dr. Faber, a specialist in neural/fascial therapy, explained to the patient that surgery and injury frequently produce adhesions of tissue and narrowing of the blood vessels leading into the places of trauma. Narrowed blood vessels cause eddy currents of the fluids surrounding the tympanic membrane and other ear structures. The result from such eddy currents is a roaring, buzzing, or ringing sensation—the tinnitus—often present with some loss of hearing.

Dr. Faber described the tinnitus condition to Mrs. Foster in this way: "It's like stepping on a garden hose and causing narrowing at a single spot. The crimping of a hose as the water rushes through causes a swirling of the flowing water through the hose. The swirling hits against the sides of the hose to produce variable decibles of noise. The same mechanism is possible in the body's own blood vessels, including those of the head. Those constrictions being near to the ear will be heard as a tinnitus. When one is fatigued, the ringing or rushing sound becomes louder inside the head."

Learning of the tinnitus mechanism and being told of neural/fascial therapy, Mrs. Foster just did not know if she wanted the proposed treatment. She was frightened of injections and wanted no semblance of extra discomfort. Dr. Faber suggested that she think about what he had explained and return sometime in the future if she decided to engage in the treatment. Two months later, Maria Foster came back to the Milwaukee Pain Clinic ready to receive neural/fascial therapy.

Using a tiny dental gauge needle, Dr. Faber carefully applied the injections to the precise areas needing injections for the neural/fascial procedure. Immediately following the treatment, Dr. Faber rubbed his fingers together near to Mrs. Foster's left ear. She could distinctly hear the slight friction rub and was excited that the ringing was gone, as well. It stayed gone, too. The series of injections were administered to Maria Foster in August 1989. Checking with the patient over a year later, she reports that the corrected tinnitus and restored hearing is permanent.

Basic Laws of Biology

Maria Foster's problem was brought on by a disturbance in the structure of her middle ear. First it occurred from the pathology of cholesteatoma. Then the structure was damaged additionally by resultant scarring from ear surgery. Dysfunction had to follow.

There is a basic law of biology:

"STRUCTURE DETERMINES FUNCTIONS."

Stated another way:

"STRUCTURE IS THE MASTER CONTROLLER OF FUNCTION."

Correct function cannot exist or even allow for any function that's adequate without undisturbed structure. When blows, hits, falls, crashes, bruises, and other traumas occur to some area of the body the shapes of cells comprising tissues may be changed (see illustrations #4, #5, and #6.)

The injection technique of neural/fascial therapy into scars or other injured areas actually perform a type of bloodless surgery. The precise adhered layers of cells and tissues are loosened and separated from underlying tissues.

This is the reason that neural/fascial therapists witness immediate improved drainage of fluid, extended range of motion, and much better function in patients with the application of their techniques.

Something else to consider—another rule:

"ALL LIFE IS MOTION."

If a part of the body is abnormally hard, tight, doesn't move, is stuck in place, and generally is abnormal, this is a sign of some health problems being present. The tissue-normalizing effect of neural-fascial therapy, massage, manipulation, or the application of physical medicine may be valuable to restore motion to the body part.

Then there is a third law of biology:

"CALCIFICATION CAUSES LOSS OF RANGE OF MOTION."

Calcium leaks out of the blood, bones and some other tissues when there is an injury or imbalance. It goes to stress areas as a splinting or protective agent. There are known accepted situations in which calcification occurs. Any trauma situation that takes place to an individual causes the body to produce calcification at the site of that trauma. One of the few true physical laws in medicine that is recognized by all scientists and physicians is Wolfe's Law, the fourth rule, which states:

"BONES RESPOND TO STRESS BY MAKING MORE BONE."

Wolfe's Law implies: If the body is having a difficult time, it must send the hardest, firmest material it can muster to help support the body's troubled area. Calcium, the chief component of teeth and bone, is as hard as anything the body can produce. Not only do bones form spurs due to calcium being laid down on them and in them but all tissues under stress get calcified, as well. This calcification causes less motion to be available and less function to be achieveable. Then another truth is:

"BIOCHEMICAL STRESS CAUSES CALCIFICATION."

In describing cancer and other degenerative diseases, the textbooks of medicine are loaded with references on how tissues, cells, organs, and other body parts become calcified when biochemcial imbalance of illness takes place. If calcified tissues don't have the blood flow or the motion required in nature, they don't function as do normal tissues because of biochemical disruption. As another rule taken next:

"MENTAL STRESS CAUSES CALCIFICATION."

Hans Selye, M.D., Ph.D., a now deceased researcher who worked in the area of psychophysiology and other subjects, published significant findings indicating that emotional stress leads to calcification in laboratory mice.[1] Moreover, a seventh law of nature exists which says:

"CASTING AN EXTREMITY WITH PLASTER OR SOME OTHER

IMMOBILIZING MATERIAL CAUSES CALCIFICATION."

When a person with an injured limb is casted or splinted, calcium develops in the immobilized areas. Also for anyone who is inactive, as for instance, a hospitalized patient, stiffness sets in and calcium develops in the tissues.

When there is inactivity in joints, calcium leaks out of the blood and bones and deposits in the tissues, causing stiffness and loss of range of motion. Then we should consider the rule that states:

"CALCIFICATIONS MAY BE CONSIDERED AS IF THEY ARE SCARS."

As a defense to stress, all calcifications produce a hardening in the tissues. Still, a problem exists from the laying down of calcium: The calcification creates this hardening at the expense of decreased motion, blood supply, and waste drainage. The effect is the onset of less function and the development of more pain. Then there is the ninth truism that says:

"MUSCLE SPASM CAUSES LOSS OF MOTION."

Since muscles are connected to tendons which cross the joints, increased tension on the muscles must cause a loss of motion in the joints. The muscle spasm may be secondary to the presence of injury, subluxation, and dislocation, plus there are nerve, ligament, and/or other dysfunctions which of themselves could be a primary source of disturbance. Consequently, a tenth rule follows:

"EDEMA, TISSUE SWELLING, AND BLOOD VESSEL PATHOLOGY BRING ON LOSS OF MOTION."

Increased fluid in the tissues can produce loss of motion which arises from injury, disrupted blood vessels, and blocked lymphatic flow. Weakened blood vessels may leak fluid out into the tissue spaces so as to cause swelling and loss of motion. Blood vessel clots or atherosclerotic vessel disease may also be the source of blockages that can cause fluid to accumulate in the tissues. Another biological truth says:

"JOINT DYSFUNCTION CAN CAUSE LOSS OF MOTION."

If a joint possesses pathology such as arthritis, worn or torn cartilage, unstable ligaments, or ripped tendons, such problems can lead to loss of motion. Furthermore, the joints can be out of place and result in loss of motion because of improper alignment of the structure. So, it evolves into a twelfth law:

"NERVE DYSFUNCTION CAN GIVE RISE TO LOSS OF MOTION."

Dysfunction of physiology in the brain, spinal cord, or peripheral nerves can cause loss of motion. A focus of pain in or on the body may be detected by an afferent nerve which sends its signal to the spinal cord. In the cord it travels to the brain and through an efferent nerve which will bring about a contracture of the tissue in the focus area. This increased nerve tone produces a loss of motion. All doctors recognize that

"INFECTIONS CAN CAUSE LOSS OF MOTION."

By various mechanisms, infections may be manifested by pain, inflammation, swelling, and loss of motion. As with infection, other forms of disability produce restrictions, such as:

"DEFORMITY PRODUCES LOSS OF MOTION."

If structures have enlarged, worn themselves down, failed to grow, or have shrunk, an obvious lack of motion may be observed. In effect, then, another law in biology is that

"COMBINATIONS OF ALL THE SOURCES OF MALFUNCTION AS STATED ABOVE CAN CAUSE LOSS OF MOTION."

Multiple small defects from the listing of these fifteen biological laws that we have offered can add together and produce a major defect which results in losses of motion. Moreover, there are a few more causes of such loss such as upset emotions, body toxins, and more. Until now, medical science had no way to counter these biological laws, but we fortunately have one more rule to add:

"NEURAL/FASCIAL THERAPY LOOSENS THE CALCIFICATION FOR RESTORATION OF FUNCTION."

The precise application of injections of anesthetic solution into the adhered areas of pathology may bring on immediate return of function, range of motion, and relief of pain. The Milwaukee Pain Clinic and Metabolic Research Center has collected over three dozen videotapes of people who have experienced a rapid therapeutic response—literally instant pain relief—of kidney pain, knee pain, hip pain, finger contractures, chest pain, and numerous other problems. The before and after video footage is available for viewing by any interested party.

This Is an Informational Text Only

In this book's text material you are learning how signs and symptoms are eliminated quite effectively for nearly every source of chronic pain on a regular basis by the trained and skilled physician's use of neural/fascial therapy techniques. Yet, "trained and skilled" are the keys to successful neural/fascial treatment. Both authors declare that such training and skill should be verified by the patient before he or she accepts the administration of neural/fascial therapy.

Furthermore we state that all of the information provided here comes from physicians, dentists, and other health professionals who utilize neural/fascial therapy in practice, along with case histories supplied by them and their patients, or from reference texts and clinical journal articles produced by such health professionals. This book is informational only and should not be considered as a substitute for consultation with a duly-licensed doctor. Any attempt to diagnose and treat illness or disability should come under the direction of your physician. To the best of the co-authors' knowledge and belief, all of the medicines, drug products, techniques, and other health care information referred to herein are legal. Neither of the authors have any interest, financial or otherwise, with any of the technique developers, product manufacturers, distributors, retailers, or other providers of any of the services, medicines, drugs, nutrients or other items referred to herein.

The above few paragraphs should be taken as a disclaimer against loss or damage in the event the reader makes use of the information learned in this book. No guarantee is given or implied by educational information or teaching methods supplied by this book.

Chapter Seven

TEST YOURSELF FOR SCAR INTERFERENCE FIELDS

Twenty-three-year-old Mary F. Wilcox, the newly-hired secretary for a small law firm in Anchorage, Alaska, had been ailing for six months with a pain in her right hip. It caused her to limp with a kind of "sailor's rolling gait." She consulted a traditionally-practicing orthopedic surgeon who diagnosed Mary as having trochanteric bursitis—inflammation of a sac of fibrous tissue filled with fluid and located on the upper and outer area of her right thigh bone. The orthopedist injected the site with corticosteroids, which quickly caused atrophy of the tissue and resulted in Mary having a big pit form in her skin at the site of injection. The bursitis did not get any better either.

The secretary accepted the pain for a time, but it was interferring with her job performance, so she consulted a second orthopedist. This one put her on a nonsteroidal anti-inflammatory drug (NSAID) taken by mouth, but it burned up the inner lining of her stomach. She had terrible heart burn and other symptoms of indigestion from the prescription, so that the young woman was forced to stop taking those NSAID pills. Moreover, she continued to feel awful hip pain.

As it happened, one of Mary's two bosses, a young

married attorney named Mark Donaldson, was the patient of Robert Rowen, M.D., Medical Director of the Omni Medical Center in Anchorage, Alaska. Dr. Rowen had traveled to Milwaukee and taken preceptor training with this book's co-author, William J. Faber, D.O., and was well-acquainted with neural/fascial therapy. During his Milwaukee visit, under professional supervision, Dr. Rowen studied the program of local anesthetic needling, experienced the injection procedure himself, took care of patients in Dr. Faber's clinic, gave injections to them and to fellow students, learned of the benefits and possible side effects of the treatment, and became expert in its administration. Furthermore, Dr. Rowen utilized the many diagnostic procedures related to neural/fascial therapy that is standard in Dr. Faber's teaching method. Among them is applied kinesiology, a diagnostic discipline of muscle testing that is common to the wholistic movement. However, kinesiological testing it is not understood at all by the allopathic (drug-prescribing), traditionally-practicing medical community.

Applied kinesiology, developed by George J. Goodheart, Jr., D.C., of Grosse Pointe Woods, Michigan, makes use of the discovery that each large muscle relates to a body organ. A weakness in a muscle usually means that there is a problem at the energy level in the associated organ. Indeed, by treating the muscle in a variety of ways and making it strong again, Dr. Goodheart was able to improve the functioning of the organ as well.

Research and practice in applied kinesiology led wholistic doctor John Diamond, M.D. of Valley Cottage, New

York to perfect a separate but related discipline of behavioral kinesiology, an integration of psychiatry, psychosomatic medicine, kinesiology, preventive medicine, and the humanities. Diamond used the basic testing techniques of applied kinesiology but focused more on the factors in the patient's surroundings and lifestyle that raise and lower body energy. In fact, Dr. Diamond recommends that his simple testing method be used to measure impacts of the environment upon your life energy. Behavioral kinesiology advises as to what stimuli strengthen or weaken you—how your body responds to stress, posture, specific foods, emotions, and your entire social and physcial surroundings. It is based on the newly discovered role of the thymus gland in regulating body energy.

The thymus is a bilobed organ in the root of the neck, above and in front of the heart. The thymus gland is enclosed in a capsule and divided internally by cross walls into many lobules, each full of lymphocytes (white blood cells associated with antibody production). In relation to body size, the thymus is largest at birth. It doubles in size by puberty, after which it gradually shrinks, its functional tissue being replaced by fatty tissue. The thymus controls the development of lymphoid tissue and immune response to microbes and foreign proteins (accounting for allergic response, autoimmunity, and rejection of organ transplants.

During the course of his studies, Dr. Faber adapted the best features of both applied kinesiology and behavioral kinesiology, added in aspects of osteopathic medicine, and came up with his own method of kinesiological testing that he teaches to physicians who spend time with him in a preceptorship program. Subsequently, he taught the Faber form of kinesiology to Dr. Rowen, who carried knowledge of this new testing procedure to Anchorage, Alaska. Dr. Rowen's patient, Mark Donaldson, was exposed to the kinesiological testing technique in the Omni Medical Center. Thereafter, Mark showed it to Mary Wilcox, so that she could use the muscle testing on herself to determine if old scars on any parts of her body were sources of interference fields. That way, Mary could determine if neural/fascial therapy potentially administered by Dr. Rowen had a chance of working for her.

With Mark's help in performing the kinesiology test, Mary learned that she definitely was a candidate for neural/fascial therapy.

"When I evaluated her," Dr. Rowen wrote in his case report, "she had a hollowed area at the site of the steroid injection over the right greater trochanter." On detailed history, as well, Mary revealed she had undergone podiatric surgery on her left foot for a neuroma removal. The podiatric surgeon had performed the operation in his office on her right foot just three months prior to the onset of her hip bursitis. She also had an old scar on the right side of her face that was present from a local plastic surgery.

"I asked Mary, "Are you brave?" She replied, "Yes, go ahead and give me the treatment." I proceeded to administer to her scars with neural/fascial therapy, using 2 percent procaine," advised Dr. Rowen. "Upon completion of the injections, instantly she had 100 percent pain relief. It was a lightning reaction."

She returned several days later reporting that some of the pain relief had dissipated, and she was now reduced to only a 50 percent level of comfort. I repeated the scar injections twice more over the next week, and my patient experienced 100 percent comfort again thereafter. Its nearly a year now and the pain has never returned for Mary. And "the hollowed area on her hip has filled in," concluded Dr. Rowen.

How to Test Yourself for Scar Interference Fields

A kinesiological muscle test can be carried out by yourself without pain and at little or no cost. This test is performed by checking the quality of strength in the muscle being used to monitor yourself or somebody else.

The person being tested is asked by the tester to extend the arm straight out and away from the side of the body at the shoulder level. The tester then explains to the testee that the quality of the strength of the arm muscle is to be tested.

The testee must resist downward force applied by the tester. In other words, the testee should hold his or her arm strong and resistant upward against the examiner's pressure as he or she is pushing down on the arm. The force is applied for approximately one second.

Both the examiner and the testee should note the strength of this baseline test. The purpose of this first monitoring examination is to set a mental mark of how much strength is present at the baseline. It's important not to use an arm or shoulder that contains arthritis, pain, injury, or some other health problem. Such a problem would cancel the purpose of this baseline monitoring. The participants want only a good muscle to be checked, and then rechecked.

Before checking for health problems caused by something in the surroundings or in/on the testee's body, the muscle test should be conducted several times so that the tester and the testee note the quality of the arm's strength.

Testing for Health or Environmental Problems

In combination, the body and brain have proprioceptive abilities. This means that the body and brain together can focus on different parts of themselves. An individual can enhance this focusing mechanism by touching another body area with one's own hand. Obviously this gives the brain more information about that particular body area being touched. Therefore, to test an area for a health or environmental problem, place the testee's hand on the area in question.

With the testee's arm extended outwardly to the side as previously described, on the count of three the examiner should press downwardly against the arm, as the testee resists.

If the quality of resistance is less now as compared to when the testee was not touching the body area being tested, this may be considered a positive sign that there is a health problem of some type in that tested area.

Over 25 years ago, Dr. George Goodheart made the discovery of this applied kinesiology testing technique. He has lectured around the world on his newly-found discipline of health testing. One can now test for impaired nerves, joints, scars, old injuries, and other sources of pain and disabilities.

Another frequent and unique test utilized by Dr. Faber is to apply kinesiological testing in the light and in darkness. If his patient displays weakness in the dark, it suggests a seasonal affective disorder (SAD) which may be causing depression, sensitivity to artificial light, sensitivity to sunlight, and lack of energy. He has found that about 50 percent of those patients visiting the Milwaukee Pain Clinic has this SAD condition. The curative treatment is exposure to sunlight for a minimum of 20 minutes per day and/or the ingestion of pineal gland substance (containing melatonin) to assist one's own pineal gland.

The pineal gland is a pea-sized mass of tissue attached by a stalk to the posterior wall of the third ventricle of the brain, deep between the cerebral hemispheres at the back of the skull. It secretes the hormonelike substance melatonin.[3]

Conditions Under Which Kinesiological Testing is Conducted

Kinesiological testing has its own mystique. It can be rather intriguing and certainly may be used for purposes of entertainment—something like a magic act. But Dr.

Goodheart's applied kinesiology and Dr. Diamond's behavioral kinesiology are not equivalent to some night club performance; rather they are reputable medical disciplines made use of by many physicians who practice holistic and biological forms of medicine. The usual drug-oriented, establishment-type doctor doesn't know how to apply kinesiology; in fact, it's likely that he or she is ignorant of this valuable diagnostic discipline altogether. To get around to looking for other, nontoxic, more natural methods of healing, it takes disillusionment with the large number of failures met by application of pharmaceutical agents in standard medical practice. Surely the application of kinesiological testing requires medical enlightenment to employ it as a routine part of health care practice. The exclusive prescribers of drugs usually are not so enlightened.

You can use this procedure for yourself, but there are conditions under which kinesiological testing is conducted. They are the following:

1. The tester and testee must be serious about the test and not wish to use it as a stage-show.

2. The person being tested must be open-minded and express a desire to have the test performed.

3. The test results are used by a health professional only in addition to the taking of a patient health history, physical examination, laboratory tests, X-ray examination, and other facts relavent to the patient's illness or injury. Such muscle testing with kinesiology is not meant to stand alone as the sole method of arriving at a diagnosis.

4. Kinesiological testing should be considered

experimental and investigative.

Idiosyncracies Connected with Kinesiological Testing

Inasmuch as muscle testing with applied or behavioral kinesiology is an inexact method, certain idiosyncratic tendencies of the method exist. Therefore, if employing this self-testing procedure on your own, you should be aware of the following two factors:

A. People who are quite strong or inordinately weak can be difficult to test with the kinesiological method.

For these more difficult testees, a Japanese physician, Dr. Omura has recommended the "O"-ring test. In this examination, the testee makes an O with the thumb and first (index) finger similar to the "OK" sign. The examiner then tests the testee's strength by pulling apart his or her thumb and index finger and noting the resistance. If the individual's strength is overly weak or strong, the thumb and second (middle) finger are used to make an O-ring. The test is repeated to have a moderately strong test to use as a baseline. If this second set of fingers are inadequate, the additional fingers may be employed to see if they will provide an acceptable modicum of strength.

B. In the case of a young child or an elderly individual in which kinesiological testing becomes invalid because strength is too weak to accurately monitor, electroacupuncture testing according to Voll, leg length, cranial rhythm, and/or other scientific techniques may be used instead.

We cannot and do not assume any liability for any reader using the information included here for purposes of diagnosing himself/herself or for injury resulting from application of the education acquired from us and employed for self-help at home. The practice of medicine is best done on a one-to-one basis between physician and patient. However, occasionally people do help themselves if they know what to do, and this self-help procedure is the topic of Chapter Six. This next chapter offers two primary methods of self-administered assistance for attaining more mobility with less pain by offsetting scar interference fields.

Chapter Eight

HELP YOURSELF TO OVERCOME SCAR INTERFERENCE FIELDS

The function of scars is often misunderstood. Scars are a necessary and important part of the healing process. Without the ability to make scars one would die either of bleeding or of other complications such as infection.

A scar is the mark left on the skin or other tissue after a wound or sore has healed. Scars are made up of fibrous material called cicatrix. The cicatrix replaces the damaged tissues of a healing wound with newly created connective tissue. Although most small scars fade as time goes by, some cicatrix may leave minor or unsightly permanent marks on the skin.

Scars on the inside of the body rarely give trouble; yet, occasionally adhesions occur when scar tissue sticks to neighboring tissues and organs, sometimes interfering with normal function.

Although cicatrix is needed by the body, the scars themselves that develop must also heal well or other problems may arise. While they may rupture, the more common mechanical problem with scars is that one or more may cause the body's shell to grow too tight. When this occurs layers of tissue are not able to move freely. The result for a victim of scarring may be pain, numbness, or loss of function.

Many times a connection between the loss of function and the scar won't be apparent. Nonetheless, scars can be a main cause of loss of function and pain in a part of the body that is remote from the location of the affecting scar.

The Balloon Patch Again

Earlier in this book we compared scarring of the skin to patching a balloon. Our allusion came from James Carlson, D.O. of Knoxville, Tennessee. Dr. Carlson explained to us that if you patch a ballon, the thickening caused by the addition of the patch to the balloon's outer wall controls the entire shape of that balloon as it is blown up to expand. The patch exerts tension which causes a pulling or tightness. Such tightness ultimately alters and controls the entire shape of the balloon.

In a similar manner, Dr. Carlson advises, when a person has a scar and then gains weight, the probability of that scar causing dysfunction increases, because the connective tissue fascia of the body is similar to the walls of a balloon. The scar, or patch, is taking up room on the wall or skin of the body.

George Goodheart, D.C. of Grosse Point Woods, Michigan describes scarring's effect on the body in another way. In his description, Dr. Goodheart explains that if muscle, tendon, skin, or fascia become tightened in one area, the tightening can result in problems in other, even remote areas of the body at a distance from the scar. The tightening will probably result in loss of motion, contracture, loss of strength, abnormalities in sensation, and chronic pain.

Dr. Goodheart's concept includes the following analogy: If a tailor pulls down hard on the right side of the shirt that you are wearing, this action makes it more difficult for you to raise your right arm. Treating your right arm with physical therapy or some other remedy would do little to relieve the decreased range of motion of the right arm as long as the tension is exerted on your shirt. Loosening the tension on your shirt's hem, however, does, effectively, produce a marked increase in the range of motion of your right arm, because you then are getting to the cause of the problem and fixing it (see illustration #8).

Dr. Goodheart further suggests that scars can cause multiple alterations of nerves, lymph, blood, and nutrient flow not only to the scar but also to more remote areas of the body such as fingers and toes.

The staff of the Milwaukee Pain Clinic and Metabolic Research Center often see patients whose areas along the back are very sensitive—even to light touch—after these people have undergone back surgery. In many of the sensitive people, Dr. Faber uncovers that the surgical scar has been causing much of their extreme pain and sensitivity. Fortunately, injection treatment with the dental-type anesthetics such as procaine, lidocaine, XylocaineTM and/or other chemical members of the "caine" family injected into the scar, connective tissue, and nerves frequently results in a marked decrease in the patient's pain and also brings about an improvement in his or her function.

The improved function results from the injected local

anesthetics causing immediate resolution of one or more scars' interference fields. As we discussed in Chapter Three, these interference fields create interruptions of the normal nerve cell electrical balance. The two German physicians, brothers Walter and Ferdinand Huneke, who, in 1925, discovered this physiological attribute of local anesthetics used their own analogy to explain how the anesthetics work to produce neural/fascial therapy. They described the phenomenon of therapy as being similar to fixing an electrical short circuit. When the short is eliminated the lights go on immediately like the striking of a bolt of lightning. Thus, they named the instant pain relief that results from injection of local anesthetics under and around an individual's scars as the "lightning reaction."

How to Nearly Simulate the Lightning Reaction for Yourself

You can self-treat a problem scar in two primary ways, and in doing so it's possible to nearly simulate the lightning reaction of Huneke. The first way is quick and easy. It merely consists of vibratory massage with the fingers.

Since one of the main problems produced by a scar is adhesion of the tissues, you may vigorously rub the scar deeply in a back and forth motion. Such massage may cause you some discomfort at the time of rubbing but repeated massage vibrations with your fingers may eventually dislodge the adhesion.

You may add to the effect of massage by soothing the area with a vitamin E ointment application placed topically between the times of self-treatment. The vitamin E may be absorbed by the skin and help the scar come detached from the underlying areas. Your attempt should be dedicated to doing what the injection procedure is supposed to accomplish—nonsurgical dissection of the scar—lifting it away from its adherence to underlying tissue.

Note: This is information offered for your personal use only. It is not appropriate for an unlicensed person to act as a health professional and give massage treatment to others. There are strict laws with heavy penalties for practicing massage therapy, making a diagnosis, or giving medical-type treatment without possessing a health professional's state license.

The second approach to helping yourself with overcoming scar interference fields is with the use of particular exercises that concentrate on body parts and locations which exhibit scarring. Yet, here, again we must offer a warning: For most people, proper exercise presents no danger to health. To minimize risk, however, we recommend that all persons over age 30 consult a physician before attempting vigorous exercise. Inform the doctor of your intentions so he can focus on those tests and health history questions that relate to coronary heart disease or some other possible problem which may arise from exercising.

When you exercise, always be sensitive to any physical symptoms that could indicate health problems, particularly any abnormal heart action, chest pain, or dizziness. If these occur, stop exercising immediately and consult a physician.

In the sections that follow, we shall describe specific exercises for the particular region or organ that may possess the scar or adhesion which is causing too tight a body shell and producing some limitation of motion, loss of function, and/or chronic pain.

Exercises for Head, TMJ, Neck, and Myofascial Pain

Certain destructive habits followed in daily living—drinking coffee, cola, liquor, and black tea, and eating chocolate and highly sugared foods—may give rise to pain in the head and neck. Eliminating such poor eating habits may break up the cycle of pain-spasm-pain that leads to muscle disability, small joint arthritis, joint malfunction in the head and neck, spinal pain, and jaw-joint pressure. For head pain, neck pain, myofascial pain, and temporomandibular joint (TMJ) syndrome, for instance, excellent self-help procedures include:

1. Eliminate the imbibing of stimulating beverages for at least two weeks (as a test) and continue the abstinence if this healthy practice proves effective for you.
2. Practice relaxation, meditate, or listen to quiet music before retiring.
3. Both morning and night, perform the following jaw exercises:

    A. Sit sideways in front of a full-length mirror; hold a smaller mirror so that you can see your profile.

Note alignment of your shoulders, neck, and head. Prevent your head from dropping forward. Prevent your shoulders from rounding forward. Sit straight at all times, tuck in the chin like a soldier. Throw shoulders back and upward.

B. When reading a book, as an ideal distance for reading attempt to hold the book's center just 16 inches from your eyes.

C. For the TMJ, with the mouth open an inch, place your fist in front of your lower jaw and try to jut the jaw forward against the immovable fist.

D. Place your fist on one side of the jaw and similarly thrust your lower jaw against the fist. Do this on the other side. Finally place your fist beneath the lower jaw and thrust against it. In each instance hold the thrust for at least 10 seconds and repeat six times in each direction. Perform the exercise morning and evening.

E. Specifically for the neck: Turn your head to the left and back to the center. Turn your head to the right and back to the center. Drop your ear toward your shoulder. Drop your ear toward the other shoulder. Look up. Look down. Repeat these simple exercises whenever you get a chance, but do them a minimum of three times daily.

F. Do these head, neck, and TMJ exercises every day.

Exercise Self-Treatment for Myofascial Pain

Seen as one of the common causes of chronic lower back pain, myofascitis is inflammation of muscle and the fibrous coverings of muscle and surrounding ligaments. Myofascial pain is brought on by continual straining of the muscle, sudden muscle trauma, or scar formation in muscular fibers around the neck, upper back, and shoulders. It can be treated at home with stretching, a change of habits, and massage. Be sure to investigate any habitual tasks or postures that may repeatedly stress muscles, because successful self-treatment depends on modifying or eliminating such perpetuating factors. Drugs are seldom necessary in the treatment of myofacial pain.

Samuel A. Skootsky, M.D., assistant professor of medicine at the University of California, Los Angeles, School of Medicine, says: "It sounds simplistic, but it's actually very important in myofascial pain syndromes to sit up straight and maintain good posture. Bad posture contributes significantly to the pain." "If you discover a discrepancy in your leg lengths, corrective shoes may be required. We recommend that you should perform stretching exercises in a hot shower if you're attempting to self-treat myofascial pain."

Exercises for Painful Shoulders

Shoulder pain is second only to back pain as a cause of time lost from work, although the shoulder is not often a problem before age 25 or after age 65. Shoulder ailments come mostly from direct injuries in accidents, hard work, and vigorous sports such as playing rugby or when you fall on an outstretched arm and jam your shoulder joint. The following is a series of simple self-help exercies for painful shoulders:

1. <u>The shoulder pendulum exercise</u> has you start in a standing position bending from the waist with arms hanging freely.

A. Swing the arm of the painful side forward, then backward, then side-to-side.

B. Make a clockwise circle with your arm; then reverse and circle in a counter-clockwise direction. Swing your arm, not your body.

C. Repeat five times in each direction.

2. <u>The assisted shoulder flexion exercise</u> has you start in a standing or lying position with a pole or cane held in both hands.

A. With straight elbows lift the pole over your head and as far back as possible.

B. Then, bending the elbows, try to bring the pole down in back of your head.

C. Return to the starting position.

D. Relax.

E. Repeat five times daily.

3. <u>The wall-climbing exercise</u> has you start standing while facing a wall.

A. Using the hand of the painful side, walk two fingers up the wall, stepping closer as you climb higher.

B. Relax.

C. Repeat five times daily.

4. <u>The shoulder shrug series</u> has you start in a standing or sitting position.

A. Pull the shoulders up toward your ears.

B. Press the shoulders down to make a long neck.

C. Let the head drop forward, rounding the back, and bring your arms forward with the back of your hands together.

D. Lift the head, stretch the arms back with your thumbs up to stretch the chest.

E. Repeat five times daily.

Exercises for Painful Knees

The following exercises help you to increase flexibility in the painful muscles that control your knees. If you are just starting an exercise program, repeat each exercise only five times and hold the stretch for a count of 10. As you become more fit, increase the exercise's repetitions.

1. To stretch the hamstring muscles, sit on the floor and extend one leg to the side. Place the other with the knee bent and set with the sole of your foot against the inside thigh of the straight leg.

A. Grasp the foot or ankle of the straight leg with your hands and slowly lower your head to your knee.

B. Lean forward from the hips with a straight back.

C. Try to keep your buttocks on the floor.

D. Reverse the position of your legs and repeat the exercise.

2. An alternative exercise for stretching the hamstrings has you stand with one foot on a bench or chair.

A. Keep both legs straight and place your hands on your hips.

B. Slowly bend forward and try to touch your head to the knee of the raised leg.

C. Hold your back straight, and place your hands on your hips.

3. The cat-stand exercise stretches the hamstring muscles in both legs at the same time.

A. From a standing position, squat down and place your palms on the floor, and flex both your hips and knees.

B. Then slowly straighten your knees while keeping your palms on the floor.

C. As you extend your knees, contract your abdominal muscles.

Don't worry if you cannot completely straighten your legs while performing the cat-stand exercise. This exercise will still stretch the hamstrings even with the knees slightly bent. (In fact, the cat-stand exercise also works well to put stretch on the lower back. So if you feel any stress on your lower back you may want to bend your knees slightly.)

4. The quadriceps stretch is done while lying on your side or standing up; however, standing up requires a bit more balance, and you might need to hold on to the back of a chair.

A. Lie on your left side and support your head in your left hand.

B. Grasp the ankle of your right foot with your right hand and pull your foot toward your buttocks.

C. Keep your right hip forward, and be sure to keep your body in a straight line and your left leg straight.

D. Repeat the exercise while lying on your right side.

Elbow, Wrist, and Hand Exercises Against Pain

The term "tennis elbow" is often applied to any elbow pain; but, in fact, it refers to a group of soft-tissue disturbances that lie outside the elbow joint. "Golfer's elbow" is a term applied to pain and tenderness of the inner side of the elbow. Both problems arise from injury, and may be an accumulation of many strains or one single event.

1. The mobilizing exercise for an elbow assists in alleviating pain for the tennis player's plight.

A. Place your arm on the kitchen table. Grasp a 2-pound weight and allow your hand to hang over the edge of the table, first palm down and then palm up.

B. In each position let the weight pull your hand down below the table.

C. Then raise it back up.

D. Repeat 50 times palm down, then palm up for one to two minutes twice daily.

2. The forearm stretching exercise for an elbow assists in alleviating pain for the golfer's plight.

A. Stand facing a wall.

B. Extend the involved arm toward the wall and put the palm of your hand on it, pointing fingers to the floor.

C. Slide upward until you feel a pulling sensation near the elbow.

D. Hold this position for one minute and repeat twice daily.

Bumps and lumps about the wrist may be herniated cysts called ganglions, and others may be benign tumors composed of fibrous connective tissue called fibromas. These growths may set up interference fields and promote pain in a place on the body remote from the growths themselves.

Carpal tunnel syndrome strikes the wrist, as well. It is a compression of the median nerve as it enters the palm of the hand so as to cause pain and numbness in the index and middle fingers and weakness of the abductor muscle of the thumb. Hand and wrist exercises may be effective to relieve pain and poor function when done for yourself at home on a steady basis.

1. The carpal-tunnel stretch is performed with the fingers straight.

A. Press the fingers of the affected hand against your other forearm with maximum force.

B. Slowly flex the involved wrist and hold that position about five seconds.

C. Be careful to keep the wrist tented at a 45-degree angle.

D. Return to the starting position.

E. Relax.

F. Repeat three times in succession every hour throughout the day, as feasible.

2. For wrist strengthening and reduction of pain,

grasp an 8-pound weight.

A. Rest your arm upon a table with the wrist hanging over the edge, palm down.

B. Raise the weight as high as possible without lifting the arm from the table.

C. Perform for 10 repetitions with increases in the weight and the repetitions on a steady schedule.

3. To flex the palm and cause it to stretch away the pain, place the fingers on a table, palm down.

A. While pressing the finger pads into the table, slowly draw the palms up, thus stretching the ball of the hand.

B. Do this slowly and to maximum tolerance.

C. Hold 10 seconds; repeat five times.

4. To strengthen the fingers and exercise pain away, obtain a piece of elastic at least 2 or 3 inches wide. Sew a band large enough for the four fingers to be inserted. Sew at an angle to keep the band tight at the little-finger side.

A. Place the fingertips within the top of the band.

B. Keep the palms together and pull the fingers apart against the band. (The band should be snug so that the fingers cannot be drawn farther apart than one inch.

C. Repeat for one minute twice daily, holding only a second or so for each motion.

5. The thumb stretching exercise involves grasping the affected thumb with the other hand wrapped around that thumb and pulling it straight away from the forearm.

The aim of all these exercises is to achieve as close as you can get to a lightning reaction without recourse to drugs, doctors, hospitals, or other forms of necessary therapy. This is a true self-help administration to your own or a loved one's pain problem. Exercising away your personal pain is performed, of course, when you have no access to health professional care, either because it is located too far away or because you cannot afford it. That's when you'll possibly be trying for a lightning reaction on your own.

A Last Word on the Lightning Reaction of Pain Relief

As was described in Chapter Three, when interference fields are eliminated, the patient receiving neural/fascial therapy will experience a lightning reaction of pain reversal and return of full function. This "flash phenomenon" (also referred to as the "Huneke phenomenon") shows up as a dissipation of pain within seconds by means of injections of various dental-type local anesthetics.

If, as we stated earlier, in accordance with the rules of neural/fascial therapy, a local anesthetic is injected into a suspected focus of interference, and the pain in an area distant from the location of the focus suddenly ceases for a period of at least 20 hours (eight hours for dental problems), and if this same effect can be reproduced after (and if) the pain has returned, then the doctor will have triggered and the patient will have experienced a lightning reaction of permanent pain relief.[1] This is a rapid therapeutic response which offers complete and even instant freedom from pain.

In fact, instant pain relief by means of neural/fascial therapy has been established as a bonafide occurrence all over Europe, especially in the German-speaking countries. It is only now crossing into the other continents.

Nearly every pain problem on the surface of the body and a lot of them inside the body (among affected organs), as well, respond to neural/fascial therapy. In the final two chapters that follow, we will present case histories from the files of practicing American physicians who are describing how this treatment works successfully for a variety of chronic pain difficulties. The true names and locations of these contributing doctors are given so that they may be contacted for verification of their experiences. (Their patients' identities are pseudonyms to protect their privacy and to conform to rules of the medical societies in the various states.)

Chapter Nine

PATIENT SUCCESSES WITH NEURAL/FASCIAL THERAPY

While driving in New Mexico's Sangre De Cristo Mountains, on April 27, 1989, Jean Matubeck, slim, brunette, and unmarried at age 33, was responsible for a serious automobile accident. Her car was wrecked completely as was the other car. The patient, the chief saleswoman for a fancy boutique in downtown Grants, New Mexico, received emergency treatment at a local hospital directly following the accident. But then, because health and accident insurance coverage was delayed for her, she sought no further medical attention. This, despite Jean feeling neck pain, upper and lower back pain, and with the radiation of pain into both thighs.

Eventually Ms. Matubeck could stand the discomfort no longer. By May 24th she found herself forced to consult a well-reputed orthopedist in Albuquerque, New Mexico, Gerald A. Montgomery, M.D., who is medical director of the New Mexico Orthopedic Medicine and Pain Treatment Center, P.C. Dr. Montgomery uncovered that not only did Jean Matubeck feel body structure pain, she also experienced headache which was present intermittently since her several automobile injuries.

She could not return to her normal sales work because

any bending, lifting, or twisting movements such as assisting customers with dressing into new clothing aggravated her symptoms. Any sudden movements of her head and neck also caused sharp pains in the neck and upper back. On her own, Ms. Matubeck had been taking increasingly strong doses of pain medication and muscle relaxants such as ValiumTM plus anti-inflammatory medications.

In his written report to us of complications in this woman's case, Dr. Montgomery said: "Past medical history revealed periodic episodes of severe abdominal pain associated with eating certain foods. She did not tolerate alcohol because of severe episodes of abdominal pain. She had been diagnosed previously as having porphyria."

Porphyria is one of a group of rare inherited disorders due to disturbance of the metabolism of the breakdown products (porphyrins) of the red blood pigment hemoglobin. The defect may be primarily in the liver (hepatic porphyria) or in the bone marrow (erythropoietic porphyria) or both. The prominent features include the excretion of porphyrins and their derivatives in the urine, which may change color on standing; sensitivity of the skin to sunlight causing chronic inflammation or blistering; inflammation of the nerves (neuritis); mental disturbances; and attacks of abdominal pain, which was the manifestation of porphyria being experienced by Jean Matubeck.

Dr. Montgomery's physical examination of her demonstrated obvious restriction of range of motion in the neck and upper back and pain associated with movements of the neck, midback and lower back. There was increased pain reported by Jean with the doctor's putting stress on her pelvis, and she experienced some weakness when he tested the patient's right hip flexion. The remainder of his neurologic examination was negative.

Ms. Matubeck had multiple areas of tenderness at the base of the occiput (back of the skull), neck, midback and lower back. There were no neurologic abnormalities noted in her upper extremities. X-ray films demonstrated very slight scoliosis but no evidence of any acute injury.

Also on her own, Jean Matubeck had previously prevailed on her girlfriend, a physical therapist, and got her to administer a little physical therapy at the nearby rehabilitation center in Milan, New Mexico. Jean reported to the doctor that the physical therapy may have been minimally helpful.

"In view of her history of porhyria," wrote Dr. Montgomery, "I suggested that she be seen by a neurologist for evaluation and that laboratory studies be obtained." This was done.

"Her sedimentation rate was elevated at 26 mm per hour with the upper limit of normal being 20 [mm per hour]. There was no evidence of abnormalities in the porphobilinogen," assured Dr. Montgomery, and the neurologist who evaluated her did not find any evidence to suggest porphyria. One of the laboratory findings in the rheumatic profile was positive and there was, therefore, a suggestion of an underlying disease process [arthritis] in view of the elevated sedimentation rate, abnormal rheumatic disease autoantibody (anticentromere), and her history of chronic recurrent abdominal pain.

It turns out that Dr. Montgomery is one of those physicians on the cutting edge of new advancements in medicine. He is an exponent of the treatment that rids people of chronic joint, tendon, and ligament pain. It is called reconstructive therapy about which we have written previously in our broadly distributed book, Pain, Pain Go Away (published by Ishi Press International, 1990, 330 pages, quality paperback, US$12.95). Dr. Montgomery considered reconstructive therapy for Jean Matubeck but decided against it in view of the abnormalities he had identified in the screening laboratory studies. Instead, as perhaps an even better treatment program, he offered her neural/fascial therapy.

Perhaps because health and accident insurance was not covering her medical costs, or for some other personal reason, Ms. Matubeck did not immediately return to Dr. Montgomery's office for treatment of her ongoing pain symptoms. She waited for a revisit until September 12, 1989. At that time she indicated to him that she was continuing to have problems and that the benefit from physical therapy she had been receiving was only temporary. Jean admitted that she was severely limiting her activities in an effort to avoid aggravation of her pain.

The woman had also begun using a home care device, the transcutaneous electrical nerve stimulation, or TENS, unit, in an effort to mask her pain. TENS devices are about the size of a personal audiocassette player and are carried by the individual on a belt around the waist. They include batteries and wires with electrodes that deliver an extremely low, pulsed direct current to the skin in the area of pain. They cost about $700 apiece and have been employed for self-care over 20 years. Application of the devices resulted from the belief that counterstimulation of the nervous system could modify perception of pain, like rubbing a bump on the head. Also it's thought that the self-treatment devices' low-frequency, high-amplitude electrical stimulation could raise the level of opiate-like substances, endorphins, in the spinal fluid. Little clinical evidence exists on the machines' effectiveness.

Upon his reexamination, Dr. Montgomery saw that Jean Matubeck's physical condition was essentially unchanged except that she demonstrated multiple sites of tenderness in the neck, midback and low back. The orthopedic medical doctor again discussed injection therapy with the neural/fascial technique but the woman again put off having this corrective care. In fact, she left the New Mexico Orthopedic Medicine and Pain Treatment Center for an extended period without any explanation until she found her discomfort absolutely unbearable.

Then Ms. Matubeck returned on December 15th and confessed to feeling totally miserable. On a 0 to 10 scale with the pain nonexistent at 0, she reported that her pain at the start of the day was at a level of approximately 6. By the end of the day's work in which she performed bending and lifting activities, her pain was easily hitting her hard at the number 10 level. "I can't stand it anymore," Jean cried.

Again Dr. Montgomery checked her and this time

found that pain was located primarily in the right lower back. "The patient indicated that she would like to try the injection therapy," he wrote. "She was placed in the prone position and the sites of tenderness clearly marked. She was most tender over the right iliolumbar ligament. The skin was thoroughly prepped and she was injected with 4 cc of lidocaine without preservatives. The patient was then reassessed.

"She indicated that following that injection her pain was relieved by at least 50 percent. Other sites of tenderness were also injected in the lower back," said Dr. Montgomery. "The patient returned on December 18, 1989, advising that she was feeling much better. She demonstrated that she was able to bend more comfortably although she still described a sensation of posterior "pulling" in the thighs. She told me that there was some soreness the day following her injection but within 48 hours her pain was significantly improved and the improvement persisted.

"On January 5, 1990, I received a telephone call from the patient advising me that she had visited family in California and decided to remain there. [The saleswoman had no relatives or other attachments to Grants, New Mexico, and poor work performance at the boutique caused no loss to her employers by her leaving.] She reported that she was continuing to feel better and asked for names of other physicians in the area who could provide additional neural/fascial therapy. I referred her to a fellow advocate of this injection procedure who was nearby to her California city," concluded Dr. Montgomery. (See Appendix I, for a list of American physicians administering neural/fascial therapy.)

Incidentally, if Jean Matubeck had not moved from the vicinity of Albuquerque, New Mexico, Dr. Montgomery writes: "My plan in this case would be to continue the injection therapy on a weekly or alternate weekly basis using the lidocaine or procaine as long as the patient was noting continued progress. I anticipate that she may require six to eight sessions more of neural/fascial therapy."

Neural/Fascial Therapy for Dysfunctional Internal Organs

The late Harold C. Walmer, D.O., of Elizabethtown, Pennsylvania had treated himself with neural/fascial therapy over 30 years ago. Dr. Walmer, an osteopathic physician and surgeon of national repute, was a Diplomate of Medical Acupuncture, a Diplomate of the American Board of Chelation Therapy, a Fellow of the American Osteopathic Academy of Sclerotherapy, and a founding member of the American Association of Orthopaedic Medicine.

Dr. Walmer wrote: "More than 30 years ago, prior to the time I officially knew of neural/fascial therapy I had developed a severe epigastric pain [pain in the pit of the stomach] which appeared at that time by the nature of its symptoms to be due to a peptic ulcer. X-ray films were negative for stomach and pylorus pathology. The pain radiated into my chest, and I had an EKG taken (electrocardiogram) which was essentially negative—no coronary problem."

"I experienced two years of miserable pain in the epigastric area, however, with difficulty striking following meals, pain fairly constant, and unresponsiveness to manipulative therapy, all forms of physical therapy, and all forms of drug therapy," Dr. Walmer continued.

"At this time in my osteopathic medical practice I was doing a great deal of manipulation for patients of their dorsal spines in which I would use the technique of cradling the patient in my arms and then thrusting with my abdomen and chest through the patient to my hand," explained Dr. Walmer. "When I did this manipulation, the palpation of my epigastric area and the costochondral areas of my lower ribs caused me exquisite pain."

Such a repeated pain syndrome forced Dr. Walmer to reduce the number of his manipulations, modify technique, and lighten his patient load altogether. Of course, this put a big dent in his daily income from osteopathic medical practice. Therefore, aside from the constant discomfort, it became mandatory for him to try to get rid of the pain in the pit of his stomach.

Dr. Walmer says, "To obtain relief, I injected myself with a fine needle using neural/fascial therapy techniques into these tender areas. Within two treatments my pain vanished, never to recur."

In another deep organ case in which the patient was given instant pain relief, Dr. Walmer tells of the 60-year-old garden supply merchant, Austin Grossworth of Harrisburg, Pennsylvania, who had a long history of chronic obstructive lung disease. Mr. Grossworth also had developed severe abdominal pain.

"This man's lung capacity was restricted to only 20 percent of normal," writes Dr. Walmer. "Usual antacids and antispasmodics were ineffectual for him. I studied the patient with upper and lower gastrointestinal (GI) X-ray films which looked normal. Yet his pain was severe and excruciating which caused him constant abdominal misery.

"I ordered arteriograms of Mr. Grossworth to determine if he had any cardiovascular obstructions. Sure enough, arteriograms of his abdominal arteries revealed that the patient suffered with severe arteriosclerosis of the mesenteric arteries," said Dr. Walmer. "The only treatment suggested by the consulting gastroenterologist was vascular surgery of the patient's abdominal arteries." But in view of the 20 percent remaining respiratory function, no surgeon was willing to operate on this man.

"Coincidentally with his other troubles," Dr. Walmer said, "the patient developed herpes zoster (shingles) of the nerves of the 8th and 10th dorsal spine."

Herpes zoster, inflammation of the skin caused by a virus and characterized by collections of small blisters called vessicles, usually starts with pain along the distribution of a nerve often in the abdomen, followed by the development of vesicles. The disease subsides in about three weeks, though sometimes severe pain may persist for many months in the area of the affected nerve. The virus that causes herpes zoster can also cause chickenpox in children.

"To give him relief I injected these areas around the

splanchnic nerves paravertebrally with procaine," continued Dr. Walmer. "Instantly the patient stated that he had complete relief of his long time abdominal pain. This relief lasted four days and then recurred. Each time I would inject Austin Grossworth using neural/fascial therapy in the splanchnic nerves there would be instant pain relief that always lasted four days. His vascular pathology was so great that the pain never was permanently relieved because an operation for him was impossible to perform. But the patient was very grateful that neural/fascial therapy afforded him periodic relief that lasted for a time."

In a third case involving the deep internal organs, Dr. Walmer writes of a Philadelphia, Pennsylvania patient, Millie Pencoster, a licensed practical nurse, age 54, who underwent surgery for a lower intestinal cancerous tumor. The operation involved removal of Mrs. Pencoster's sigmoid colon and descending colon. The rectum was removed, as well, and the patient lived with a colostomy. She constantly complained to her surgeons, post-operatively, that she felt constant aching, gas, and awful abdominal spasm. The surgeons tried, but nothing that they gave her as treatment relieved these complaints.

Eventually Millie Pencoster made the one-hour automobile trip from Philadelphia to Elizabethtown to consult Dr. Walmer. He advises, "I saw her in consultation and felt that the peritoneal scar [from the cancer operation] might be a focus setting up this set of symptoms. Therefore, I injected her scar with procaine. There was immediate and permanent relief of all symptoms—the setting in of a lightning reaction." Mrs. Pencoster never had her GI symptoms again.

Symptoms of Memory Loss and Tinnitus Improve

A 41-year-old advertising agency executive, Rosco S. Drummond of Detroit, Michigan, consulted L. Terry Chappell, M.D., Medical Director of the Celebration of Health Center in Bluffton, Ohio, because of extreme fatigue and a feeling of light-headedness on a continuous basis. Mr. Drummond had been feeling well up until approximately six months before, but at the time of this first consultation, in January 1990, the man explained, "My spaciness is always with me. My work involves dealing directly with the agency's clients, some administrative duties, and much creativeness on the ad accounts. I can't think straight, however, and my symptoms seem to be getting worse and worse. Sometimes I'm exceedingly dizzy. My memory is definitely declining. I have a great deal of difficulty remembering names. The other day I was speaking of my family, and I couldn't even think of my little boy's name. Can you imagine that?"

Such incidents were greatly interferring with Mr. Drummond's ability to perform his work. Confidentially, Mrs. Drummond, who accompanied her husband to the Celebration of Health Center, spoke privately with Dr. Chappell and said she was afraid that Rosco was developing Alzheimer's disease. She confirmed, as well, that sometimes when he tried to explain what was happening at his advertising agency he would get lost in mid-sentence. He just couldn't formulate the thoughts into sentences. Also, he was concerned because of a strong family history of heart problems. His father, uncle, and grandfather had died from coronary thrombosis.

At first Dr. Chappell checked him carefully for heart and artery diseases such as atherosclerosis. There was none! Then he worked on diagnosing any abnormalities with Mr. Drummond's digestive processes and to identify some food allergies. There were a few problems there to treat. By avoiding the foods causing reactions, Rosco was somewhat improved, but all of his mind symptoms persisted, at least to a greater or lesser degree. After a couple of months of basic nutritional therapy, Rosco was still complaining of his head spinning, a vertigo, a feeling that he might faint any time, and a sense of floating in outer space.

With a return to history-taking, Dr. Chappel elicited from the patient that he had previously sustained a head injury on his forehead while riding a motorcycle in his young adult years. There was a small scar from the accident remaining in that area just above the left eyebrow. He also had a barely visible scar over his right eyebrow that had occurred when he fell from a tractor twelve years earlier. It was during this second session of putting his complaints on the record that Dr. Chappell learned that Rosco Drummond had some subtle hearing loss which seemed to get worse when he was exposed to recurrent loud sounds. More than that, he also admitted to being annoyed by a constant low-decibel ringing in the ears—tinnitus—which the man just had accepted as part of approaching middle-age and living in such a highly industrialized city as Detroit.

Dr. Chappell decided that his patient was a prime candidate for neural/fascial therapy with lidocaine diluted in normal saline. He injected Mr. Drummond's scars on his head and also around both ears and in the occipital area at the back of the head. Dr. Chappel writes in his case report, "Instantaneously Rosco felt better. He no longer had dizziness. The tinnitus (or ringing) in his ears was dramatically improved. He reported that all the colors in the room seemed brighter and that he felt much more alert and had more energy."

The physician had his patient return one week later. About 50 percent of the improvement that Rosco had experienced at the last visit remained. "He also felt that his breathing was better and that his sinuses had improved," Dr. Chappell said. Therefore, he reinjected those areas, with similar results immediately appearing, and this time the effects lasted permanently. The patient experienced a lightning reaction, and his troubles departed forever.

"His confusion did not return," said Dr. Chappell. "He improved to the point where he felt at least as good as he had a dozen years before when he began working at the advertising agency but before he fell from the tractor. Not only could he remember all the names of his clients and suppliers now, but he remembered all the details of their accounts in great detail." Rosco S. Drummond's Alzheimer-like symptoms had disappeared.

Correction of Sciatica and Migraine

A board certified diplomate in pain management, practicing the specialties of neurological and orthopaedic medicine, Dietrich K. Klinghardt, M.D., Ph.D., told us of his patient who suffered with sciatica. Dr. Klinghardt is medical director of the Santa Fe Pain Center in Santa Fe, New Mexico. He treated graduate student Monroe Benedict of Los Alamos, New Mexico, "a man in his mid-twenties with proven L-5 [fifth lumbar vertebra] to S-1 [first sacral vertebra] disc herniation. My patient was completely relieved of the sciatica with a total of three injections of 1 percent lidocaine into a scar in the anterior lower leg on the left side (the side on which he had his sciatica)." The neural/fascial therapy permanently eliminated the sciatic problem.

Dr. Klinghardt also advised that he cleared up a patient's severe case of chronic, severe, ongoing migraine headaches. The poor woman, Rosemary Hendricks, a homemaker, age 48, living in the little New Mexico town of Las Trampas, was "completely relieved by one single injection into a scar overlying the right hip joint (from surgical repair of a hip joint fracture 25 years ago)."

For Phillip Joyose, a 77-year-old retired ship's captain living in Rowe, New Mexico who also had a repeating migraine, Dr. Klinghardt writes: "It was completely relieved by a total of two injections into his tonsils.

"I have an endless number of cases such as these by now. Neural/fascial therapy is the most striking and elegant technique to resolve chronic pain. It is a technique I believe that every physician in the United States of America should be aware of. In West Germany, it has become the leading modality in the treatment of pain. It is hard for me to understand that this treatment modality is not more known by now here in the USA," ponders Dietrich K. Klinghardt, M.D., Ph.D.

Chapter Ten

POINTS TO CONSIDER ABOUT NEURAL/FASCIAL THERAPY

Neural/fascial therapy according to the German developers, the brothers Ferdinand Huneke, M.D., who died in 1966, and Walter Huneke, M.D., who died in 1974, is a holistic mechanism of pain regulation. These two medical doctors have affected the practice of medicine for the easement of pain far beyond their office address in Dusseldorf, Federal Republic of Germany. Exploration of the autonomic nervous system has been the secret of their therapy's success.

The Autonomic Nervous System

The healing stimulus of neural/fascial therapy comes from a correctly placed therapeutic substance most often consisting of some dental-type local anesthetic. It produces a response from the entire autonomic nervous system and from fascial planes whose pathways are followed by the three musketeers in physiology: homeostasis, pathology, and recovery.

The autonomic nervous system of a human being is a functional unit which includes the neurohumoral regulatory system in its overall mode of operation. The autonomic nervous system encompasses the sympathetic nervous system, the parasympathetic nervous system, and the basic autonomic neural system. This basic autonomic neural system is interstitial fluid, the soft connecting tissue which fills all organ interstices and spaces. It is composed of cells, nerves, capillaries, and extracellular fluid. The basic autonomic neural system plays the role of a communicator in the overall arrangement which enables each cell in the body to be in connection with every other cell. That's why injecting a scar in a remote part of the body corrects a problem of pain existing in a local part of the body.

As stated, the autonomic neural system is a part of the autonomic nervous system, that portion of the entire central nervous system which is of significance for the maintenance and reproduction of the particular cell structures involved. The autonomic nervous system primarily serves for control of the inner milieu of a human being. Since the control loops of the autonomic and somatic nervous systems are interlinked throughout the central nervous system, what happens in one part of the body indirectly affects every other part.[1]

The Neural/Fascial Method of Treatment

Treatment by local injection into scars, chronic ailments, impaired teeth, old injuries, and other sources of interference fields often affords the patient a restoration from pathology and the return to homeostasis.

In this treatment, the selective use of procaine, lidocaine, or another preferred member of the "caine" family is a segmental administration into the disease process. Improvement is achieved for the patient by repetitive injections which steadily increase in therapeutic effect. Eventually, repeating the injections into the responsible interference field will cure the disorder caused by it, as far as it is anatomically still possible to do so.

Ending that way in permanent correction, the final effect for the patient will likely be a lightning reaction or Huneke phenomenon. All disturbances remote-controlled from the interference field tend to disappear as they respond to simple injections with small quantities of local anesthetic that get well-placed.

The one contraindication for placing one of these injections is intraarterial administration into a blood vessel leading to the brain or into the subarachnoid space. It can have serious consequences for the patient. Therefore, proper training, operatory skill, and medical knowledge is all-important for mastery of the administering health professional. Neural/fascial therapy is an art of healing and not only a scientific discipline.

The treatment is administered in two forms:

A. As segment therapy in which concerted injections of anesthetic are given into the segmental area associated with the illness or pain.

B. As the elimination mechanism of a focal disorder in which the anesthetic agent renders it ineffective and brings on the lightning reaction. Statistics show that approximately 30 percent of previously therapy-resistant illnesses are caused by remote focal disorders.

In the patient case histories which follow, both types of treatment effects, segment therapy and focal disorder therapy, are included.

Permanent Relief of Pelvic Inflammation and Dysmenorrhea

Bertha Connelley is a 39-year-old married hair dresser living in Honolulu, Hawaii who was victimized by severely chronic pelvic inflammatory disease with multiple abdominal and pelvic adhesions documented by laproscopy. She remained addicted to Fiorinal with 1/2-grain of codeine—taken three times daily starting a week before her monthly flow—for the past several years because of her severe and constant pelvic pain and chronic dysmenorrhea. Dysmenorrhea is painful or difficult menstruation.

A hysterectomy had been recommended by her gynecologist on several occasions, but she was fearful of going under the knife. The operation would have eliminated painful menstruation by excising her uterus—no more monthly flow.

As an alternative treatment, numerous courses of antibiotics were tried but not helpful. Surgical lysis of the adhesions had been attempted, both by lapratomy and by laproscopy, but the procedures ended in failure. Bertha Connelley suffered. Her left fallopian tube and ovary had been removed in 1987 because most of the pain was localized to her left lower quadrant, and it was thought by the doctors that such a procedure offered her a chance for relief. It did not.

Instead, the pain symptoms gradually worsened until she was having difficulty walking, with pain radiating down the inside of her left thigh and from her left lower quadrant up into her left shoulder. As an additional curiosity, when Bertha raised her left arm above her head, it seemed to trigger the left lower quadrant pain. In fact, it seemed to worsen more than usual. In desperation, the woman gave serious thought to having her uterus removed, but first she decided she would go to a "pain management specialist" at the main local multidisciplinary pain clinic in Honolulu. She made the appointment.

Bertha was seizing at any way to get comfort. Because he was her gynecologist who had success with performing suprapubic para-uterine blocks with neural/fascial therapy on both sides of her pelvis one time previously, just prior to the pain clinic appointment she decided to drop in on gynecologist/obstetrician Joseph A. Brock, M.D. of Honolulu. "Could be that his injections will do me some good again. Maybe, just maybe, Doc Brock has something to offer," the woman thought aloud.

He did! Dr. Brock was using neural/fascial therapy rather extensively for dysmenorrhea and pelvic inflammation. He told Bertha Connelley about the procedure again. "At this visit, neural/fascial therapy was applied to all body scars, including ones on her wrists, forehead, and a well-healed lower abdominal transverse scar from her prior exploratory laparatomy. Two rows of quaddles [hive-like bumps that arise from injections] were raised over her left lower quadrant and carried out laterally to her side. The para-uterine, supra-pubic therapy from before was not repeated," Dr. Brock wrote to us.

Instant pain remission came upon Bertha. "Her relief was immediate, but partial, with 75 percent reduction in pain symptoms over the first four days. The pain, however, continued to diminish," said Dr. Brock, "so that by one week later, 95 percent of her symptoms had resolved, including the pain radiation down the inside of her left leg and up into her left shoulder. She was able to return to work."

As an interesting aside, two days after her consultation with Dr. Brock, Bertha kept the appointment she had made at the Honolulu pain management clinic. She was still in some pain then. The pain specialist who took her history and did the physical examination, according to Bertha Connelley, "brushed aside my remarks that I was definitely feeling better after some injections by Dr. Brock. He informed me that I was "chronic" and will just have to learn to live with the pain.' I decided, then, that I refuse to accept chronic pain as my destiny. Rather, my intent was to stay with those neural/fascial injections."

"She continued to improve," Dr. Brock said, "and by post-treatment day 22 she was totally symptom-free, off narcotic drugs, and quite happy with her result." Some months later, having experienced three menstrual cycles since receiving neural/fascial therapy, Bertha Connelley has had no more dysmenorrhea, and the inflammatory pelvic disease symptoms with radiating pains elsewhere are entirely gone.

Permanent Correction for Gall Bladder Inflammation

William C. Kubitschek, D.O. of San Marcos, California reports on Jason Kallisher, a 52-year-old colonel in the United States Army. Colonel Kallisher, with whom Dr. Kubitschek consulted one morning in May 1990, is a former Vietnam War and Korean War U.S. Army helicopter pilot who doesn't readily give into discomfort. However, this morning Colonel Kallisher was doubled over in pain when he arrived at the door of Dr. Kubitschek's office.

"Upon examination, evaluation, and vital signs analysis of the Colonel," Dr. Kubitschek informed us, "I determined that he no doubt had an acute cholecystitis."

Acute cholecystitis is inflammation of the gall bladder due to bacterial infection, causing fever and acute pain over the gall bladder area. If it's associated with gallstones and becomes chronic, it causes recurrent episodes of upper abdominal pain. Recurrent bacterial infection may be the cause, but the physical processes leading to gallstone formation may also be important.

"I carried out neural/fascial therapy on Colonel Kallisher in the 10th and 11th inner space between the ribs—with amazing results. The soldier responded within four minutes. He began to feel remarkably better and relaxed. Within ten minutes he was able to sit up and converse normally. He showed complete recovery from his acute gall bladder symptomology"

Robert Rowen, M.D. of Anchorage, Alaska also reported on the reversal of pain from a patient's cholecystitis. A railroad conductor, 48-year-old Jonathan Waggoner of Fairbanks, Alaska, was between work shifts in Anchorage when he was struck by severe gall bladder pain. At the local hospital emergency room where he went, a member of the hospital's board of directors happened to be present, and this board member also is an admiring patient of Dr. Rowen's. The hospital director actually referred Jonathan Waggoner out of his own hospital for treatment of the problem at Dr. Rowen's office.

Being struck by gall bladder pain was no surprise to Jonathan Waggoner. For seven days he had been ignoring right upper quadrant pain and previously had been told by his doctors and a surgeon in Fairbanks that he needed urgent gall bladder surgery. Interestingly, X-ray examination and scans of his gall bladder were negative, yet he was scheduled for surgery when he was to return to Fairbanks on the next train.

"In the course of evaluating him, I found that he had a large scar across the right abdomen and flank from a previous nephrectomy (kidney removal) three years before. He had had kidney cancer," Dr. Rowen wrote. "Not finding anything else to cause a dysfunctional gall bladder, I recommended neural/fascial therapy on the scar. Mr. Waggoner agreed, and it was injected by me with 2 percent procaine. His right upper quadrant pain vanished immediately and has never returned to this day—five months later. He cancelled his surgical procedure that day, from my office, and was spared a $15,000-unnecessary operation."

Corrective Treatment for the Knee

A woman who does private cleaning in people's homes, Ellen Riesdale, age 39, of Lima, Ohio was for two decades deeply involved with running. It was practically an addiction for her. However, for the past two years she had been ailing with pain on the outer aspects of her left knee. This pain gave Ellen so much trouble it not only stopped her from enjoying her pastime, it also hurt while she did her housework jobs for clients.

Having accompanied a girlfriend who was the patient of L. Terry Chappell, M.D., Medical Director of the Celebration of Health Center in Bluffton, Ohio, on visits to the Center for several months, Ellen considered consulting the doctor about her knee. It was not a decision to be taken lightly, for she was very skeptical about all doctors. She wanted to be sure that she had absolute confidence in a new physician if she decided to place herself under his care. Finally, her evaluation of Dr. Chappell allowed Ellen to present herself as a patient.

After physical and laboratory examinations, Dr. Chappell decided to do intraneural injections around the patients knee to try to free up the circulation at the nerves that were coming down the outside of her leg. The area of pain was not in the ligaments of the knee, and therefore reconstructive therapy, in which Dr. Chappell is expert (see Dr. Chappell's four case histories in Pain, Pain Go Away by

Faber and Walker, published by Ishi Press International, Inc. of Mountain View, California) was not used.

Dr. Chappell's employment of neural/fascial therapy proved highly successful. He writes: "After the first injection session, Ellen had a lightning reaction, with an immediate relief of pain. It lasted 24 hours. A second session the following week gave her total relief of pain that did not return despite her continuing to work and starting to run once or twice. Soon afterwards, she was absolutely delighted that she was able to return to regular running every morning."

Elimination of Foot and Ankle Sprain

While working at unloading a truck full of paper goods at his company's warehouse, 31-year-old Bucky Fensterhall of South Valley, New Mexico injured his right foot and ankle. He had what appeared to be a classic ankle sprain, but it did not get better even with applicaton of ice packs. Two days later, therefore, he visited the New Mexico Orthopedic Medicine and Pain Treatment Center in Albuquerque for a consultation with orthopedic medicine physician Gerald A. Montgomery, M.D.

Bucky had slipped on a wet floor exerting his foot sharply while carrying a giant box of mailing bags. The swelling, redness, and pain that came over his ankle had him in agony. He had not previously experienced such a problem, and there was no history of gout or other inflammatory arthritis for him. Dr. Montgomery saw that his patient walked with a limp, placing almost all of his weight on the unaffected side. In his report to the coauthors, the orthopedist said: "Examination of the right ankle demonstrated obvious swelling and aggravation of the pain associated with eversion of the foot and ankle. There was local tenderness present over the deltoid ligament and over the anterior aspect of the right ankle. There was also some tenderness over the dorsum of the foot along the navicular bone and the first and second cuneiform bones.

"X-ray films that I took of the right ankle demonstrated some degenerative changes at the ankle joint and at the talonavicular joint [where the ankle bone meets the foot bone], but there was no fracture. Screening laboratory studies showed a uric acid level that was at the upper limits of normal," wrote Dr. Montgomery. The slightly elevated uric acid reading indicated that Bucky Fensterhall had a tendency toward gouty arthritis."

"Following the examination, I suggested to the patient that we locally anesthetize the area of injury. [Such an injection is a technique of neural/fascial therapy.] He agreed! The sites were injected with lidocaine without preservatives and included the deltoid ligament and ligaments around the right navicular bone (at the tarsonavicular and cuneonavicular ligaments)," Dr. Montgomery said. "The patient felt significant relief." Following the injections he was instructed in exercises in a nonweight bearing position.

"The patient was seen 12 days later and reported that his ankle had significantly improved. He was able to bear full weight with walking and there was no swelling present.

There was minimal tenderness to palpation along the deltoid ligament. The patient was asked to return to the office in six weeks or sooner if there were continued problems," concluded Dr. Montgomery. "He called to report that his ankle had healed completely and that there were no restrictions. No further follow up appointment was required."

Chapter Eleven

RESOLUTION OF PAIN AND DYSFUNCTION IN THE HEAD

At age 42, Clarice Schroeder of Houston, Texas, a clerical secretary to the executive director of a charitable organization, had been victimized for twelve years by disabling frontal headaches located at the left side of her head. Ms. Schroeder, a divorced woman, had been diagnosed by means of CAT scans, magnetic resonance imaging, and many other sophisticated medical tests as having "migraines". It was common for her to be laid low even on the job and to leave her place of employment in order to find her way home to bed. Because of her frequent absenteeism and her inability to function during attacks of migraine, she had lost two jobs and one husband. Now she was in danger of being fired again.

The pain that struck with alarming regularity was blinding in nature which is characteristic of the migraine headache. Before it hit, Ms. Schroeder invariably felt nausea, queasiness, and had vomiting. An aura that preceded the pain, consisted of flashes of light in the center of her field of vision or a flickering sensation in one eye. When the aura appeared, she always had feelings of apprehension, irritability, and restlessness. They were the certain signs of an impending attack. Sensitivity to light, sweating, and disorientation were other associated symptoms. The headaches varied in frequency, sometimes they occurred every day; occasionally they stayed away for more than a week.

As an individual whose life was disrupted by frequent migraine attacks, the woman learned to anticipate onset soon enough to ward off the worst symptoms by taking aspirin, phenobarbital, or tranquilizers. Also she avoided certain foods and alcoholic beverages which seemed to be responsible for triggering the headaches. She did get some help from swallowing more potent drugs such as InderalTM, DarvonTM, and codeine, but they impaired her ability to function altogether. Since she knew that her current job was on the block, there came a time when Ms. Schroeder couldn't take anticipation of her head pain anymore. That's when she sought the services of John L. Sessions, D.O., of Kirbyville, Texas. She traveled a long way from Houston to consult him for relief.

Dr. Sessions saw Clarice Schroeder at his clinic in June, 1988. After his careful examination, he determined that her problem really came from her teeth. To clarify his diagnostic impressions, Dr. Sessions asked a nearby dentist to provide him with a full set of X-ray films of Ms. Schroeder's jaws—a panogram. It turns out that she did have an oral interference field in the form of granuloma, a degenerate mass of cells at the apex of the roots of some teeth on the left side of her jaw, especially significant was a large growth of cells at her left canine tooth. The granuloma's field of interference behaved like a time bomb in her mouth that exploded periodically in the form of disabling head pain.

What did Dr. Sessions do next? He administered two series of neuro/fascial therapy injections to the patient, including injections around the nerve roots affecting the left forehead area. Amazing though it seemed to Clarice Schroeder, she improved with just the first treatment series. The second set of injections reinforced the initial neural/fascial therapy, and she has been well since, without a single migraine headache returning for the past two years. It's not anticipated that she will have any migraine headache again.

Potential Health Problems from Dental Interference Fields

Any potential interference field may remain inactive for years, because the body's own immune defenses are intact and operating (see illustrations #13 of Chapter Two). Still, inflammation, traumatic tissue, lesions with or without visible scar formation, unresorbable foreign bodies, and degenerative processes can singularly or all of them together produce a permanent pathogenic effect. The teeth, in particular, are an area of the body either ignored or most often overlooked by health professionals, except, perhaps, dentists. Even then, most dentists have not yet recognized the changes that must be regarded as possible causes for systemic illnesses due to a person having an interference field.

Any individual with head lesions such as several dental granulomas, scars, shrapnel splinters, infected paranasal sinuses, and/or inflamed tonsils most frequently encounter interference fields. A dentist certifying that the teeth need not be regarded as a focus of the patient's illness, because the dental X-ray films show no granuloma to be present, or who reaches the same conclusion on the strength of a simple visual inspection of the oral cavity, is not offering any satisfactory or worthwhile statement. The health professional needs more education.

Eventually, that individual with the head lesion is likely to experience a lowering of his or her immunological threshold, and the interference field can then become the source of pathogenic activity. Such a lowering of the immune defense threshold may occur with some simple change in everyday circumstances, including accidents, surgery, dental-root treatment, serious illness, psychological stress, or any combination of two or more of these components. Iatrogenic factors (circumstances arising from administrations by doctors), such as the prolonged use of large doses of body regulation blockers, like corticosteroids, antibiotics, chemotherapeutic preparations, or psychotherapeutic drugs can also contribute to immune suppression.

By itself, the interference field is generally limited in extent and produces few or no local symptoms. Permanent irritation stimuli nevertheless emanate from it which continually stress the control circuits of the regulating system with outside energy and are capable of triggering remote disturbances in other parts, systems, organs, and tissues of the body.

Peter Dosch, M.D., from whose collective written work this information is derived, says that oral interference fields may affect the following body areas:

1. Sinuses: causing complaints involving the maxillary and other nasal accessory sinuses; chronic catarrh; hayfever; offensive nasal discharge; constantly blocked nose; nasal polyps; deviated septum or septal surgery; supraorbital neuralgia.

2. Thorax: causing complaints involving tuberculous processes; pneumonia; pleurisy; pleural adhesions; endocarditis; myocarditis; pericarditis; thoracic contusions still sensitive to pressure or tapping.

3. Abdomen: causing complaints involving hepatitis; cholecystitis; gastric or duodenal ulcer; dysentery; cholera; typhoid fever; pancreatitis; infantile dyspepsia; grumbling appendix; chronic diarrhea; chronic constipation; colitis; food poisoning; abdominal surgery; renal calculi; nephritis.

4. Pelvis: In women: causing complaints involving gonorrhea; pelvic inflammatory disease; vaginal discharge; dysmenorrhea; menstrual abnormalities; abortions; terminations of pregnancy;, D & C or other similar surgery; difficult deliveries such as forceps, breech, perineal tear or episiotomy. In men: causing complaints involving venereal disease; orchitis or epididymitis; prostatitis; benign prostatic hypertrophy; micturition difficulties; nonspecific urethritis; frequent nocturia.

5. Bones: causing complaints involving fractures; painful coccygeal contusion; periosteal disease; osteomyelitis; Scheuermann's disease and other aseptic necroses of bone; rib resections; surgery to fingers and toes.

6. Skin and subcutaneous tissue: causing com-

plaints involving chronically painful or itchy areas; ecthyma and other pustular skin conditions; leg ulcer; painful varicose veins; sites of earlier thromboses; recurrent skin inflammations such as neurodermatitis; torn ligaments; lacerated muscles; arterial ligatures.

7. Foreign bodies: causing complaints involving shrapnel; broken needles; glass; grains of sand; pinned bone fractures; different metals in the mouth used for dental fillings; cardiac pacemaker.

Interference Fields in Trigeminal Neuralgia

A fifty-two-year-old female physician, Gladys Moorehead, M.D., of San Francisco, who specializes in internal medicine, reported that she repeatedly suffered from severe attacks of trigeminal neuralgia after consuming small amounts of alcohol. Another name for her condition is tic douloureux. Dr. Moorehead's symptoms consisted of brief attacks of sudden severe stabbing facial pain along the course of the trigeminal (fifth cranial) nerve in the face. The stabbing pain that she experienced was momentary but recurred over periods lasting about 20 seconds, triggered by touching, a slight draft, or the application of cold water on the sensitive spot as when she washed her face. Also, her attacks were influenced not only by drinking alcohol but by seasonal changes, as well, and the trigeminal neuralgia did seem to occur mostly in the spring or autumn months, gradually increasing in frequency and severity. The absence of symptoms for Dr. Moorehead lasted weeks at a time, and then they would come on repeatedly and frequently, especially if she drank alcoholic beverages including wine or beer. These attacks were taken as evidence of the doctor having an alcohol allergy.

The physician's tic douloureux went away when a colleague administered neural/fascial therapy to her. It turns out that the wrong bite of an otherwise unsuspected dental crown was the cause. It needed to be corrected, and when it was the trigeminal symptoms never returned for Dr. Moorehead. Of course, the dentist who did the dental crown bite correction, being unknowledgeable about interference fields, doubted the validity of his mechanically corrective procedure.[2]

Chronic Inflammation of the Jaw Bone

Remote neural/fascial disturbances can be caused by inflammatory changes near the roots of teeth, which barely show on X-rays, by osteomyelitic foci, by displaced teeth, by teeth used as buttresses for bridgework and therefore subjected to excessive stress, and by radicular, paradental or follicular cysts. In cysts there is a constant decomposition of protein. This, together with the tendency of cysts to grow, is sufficient reason for their removal. The same applies to a variety of dental difficulties including odontomas, conglomerates of dental tissue, hypercementoses, and all sclerosing processes in the jaw bones. Gingivitis, stomatitis, and parodontoses produce pockets, which become sources of chronic inflammation and irritation.

A stomatitis which occurred years ago in the dental patient with no visible changes at the time can have left behind a latent interference field. It may become active at a later date by some second insulting trigger factor to the system.

The importance of osteitis in any search for an interference field is becoming more readily recognized by neural/fascial therapists. Formerly, the patient's defensive capability was suffciently intact to enable the gums to heal by themselves after a dental extraction. Nowadays, environmental and internal pollution have reduced this immune defensive capability. It's a state made worse through the routine use of antibiotics as a main contributing factor to chronic, residual osteitis. What's seen by the therapist is a persistent chronic inflammatory condition in the maxillary and mandibular bones of the patient's jaw. Their identification and evaluation need to be done on X-ray films by means of an oral panogram (full circumventing view of all teeth and gum areas of the mouth).

The dental surgeon has to think more globally than merely as an extractionist of infected or impacted teeth. The dental surgeon has an importance with regard to the pathological processes taking place in a person's body and not only in his mouth. Such an informed dentist can be an invaluable ally and not only a "narrow-gauge physician". A partnership with the physician neural/fascial therapist and the dental surgeon will be a genuine boon to the long-suffering patient who is suffering with chronic head pain and dysfunction.[4]

Spanish stomatologist Dr. Ernesto Adler calls the

wisdom teeth "teeth of misfortune" because almost all wisdom teeth, especially those out of alignment, have deep marginal pockets promoting chronic bacterial growth and inflammatory irritation. Dr. Adler observes that the real misfortune of wisdom teeth occurs after their extraction. Standard orthodox dental training teaches not to clean out (curette) the surrounding bone tissue. The result of this lack of cleansing is that bone heals over the surface of the now vacant bone socket but the infection remains. Often the unsuspecting patient experiences very littl discomfort when the osteitis (bone infection) remains in its chronic state. These areas generally escape detection when dentists employ the usual orthodox guidelines of X-ray diagnosis. The key to diagnosis is by carefully examining the patient's dental arch by means of the panorex or panoral X-ray exposure. The panoral X-ray technique utilizes a single X-ray film of the entire mouth and both jaws. Often the changes seen on this film are not sharply defined and can generally be recognized by their blurred bone structure. Too bad that this type of X-ray filming and the biological dentistry concept is not commonly used by the vast majority of dentists. Perhaps this book will enlighten some dentists who read it. The dental profession must become aware of the pivotal role its practicing members play in the overall health of their patients' body and mind.

A Child's Pathology Because of Head Trauma at Birth

"Little Joe" Mailer was brought by his parents from

Sioux Falls, South Dakota for a consultation with Dr. William J. Faber of the Milwaukee Pain Clinic and Metabolic Research Center. Little Joe's aunt Beverly and his grandmother and grandfather, who all live near to the Milwaukee greater metropolitan area, had received considerably effective results from being treated by Dr. Faber.

At one of the finer and better-known children's hospitals in the midwest, Little Joe had been diagnosed as a cerebral palsy victim, but no therapeutic program of consequence was offered. The baby's parents brought him everywhere looking for help, but none was effective. Now six years old, he remained cross-eyed, unable to hold up his head straight, experienced marked tenderness of the cervical spine (the neck), and fell down innumerable times throughout every day. He had difficulty riding his tricycle and made no attempt to swim when placed in the swimming pool at the local YMCA in Sioux Falls.

His history revealed that Little Joe was born small (a mere four-and-one-half pounds) and did not have a true vaginal delivery but was "precipitated". This means that the baby had undergone an uncontrolled spontaneous birth, known to be hazardous for an infant because of the tremendous force of of the mother's uterine contractures induced on a baby's head and neck. Small babies such as Joe were least able to withstand this type of severe contractural trauma. Subsequently, early in life Little Joe possessed huge dents in his frontal and parietal cranial bones (see photograph #1 and photograph #2.)

As the small boy grew, his parietal frontal dent

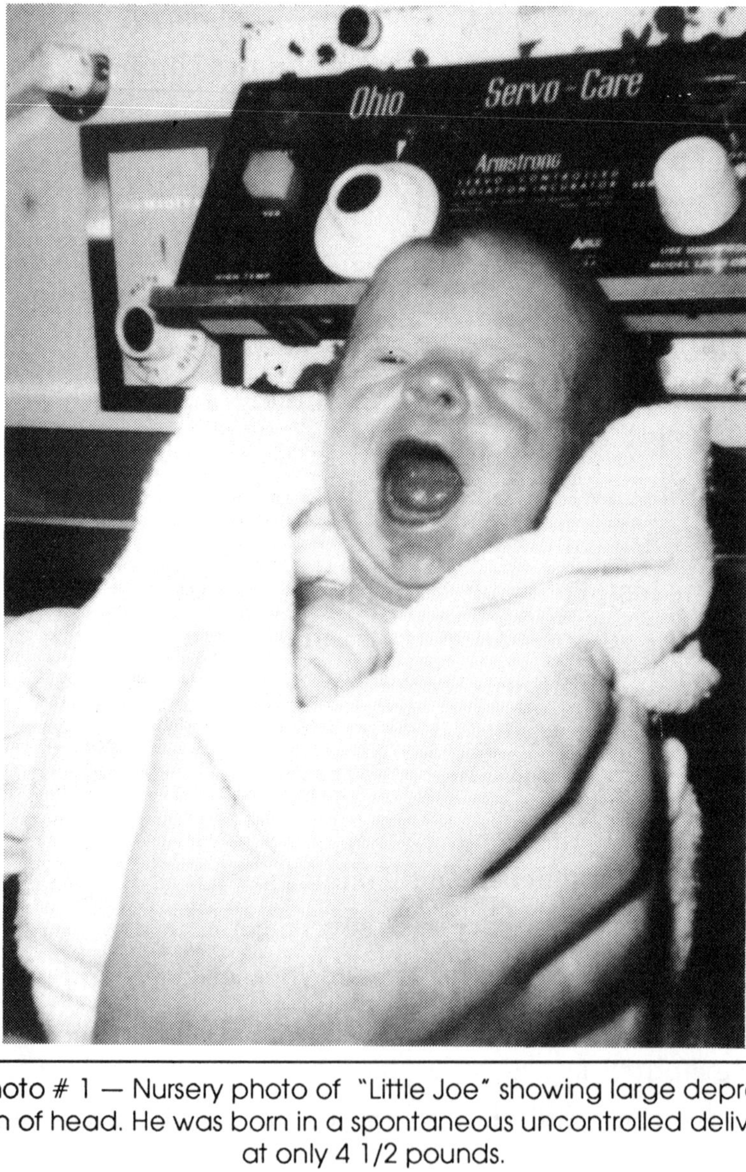

Photo # 1 — Nursery photo of "Little Joe" showing large depression of head. He was born in a spontaneous uncontrolled delivery at only 4 1/2 pounds.

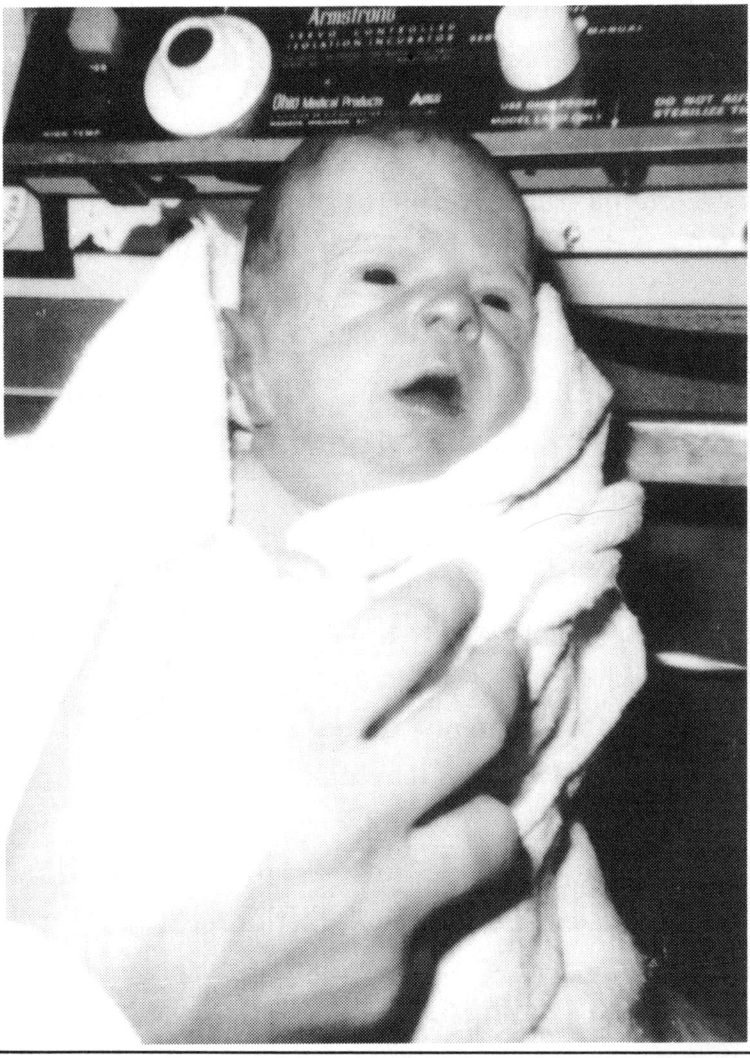

Photo #2 — Another view of "Little Joe's" head in the nursery.

worked outward, but the birthing toll became apparent in other ways, some of which have been described. He never held up his head in a straight alignment and forever tilted it to the left. He remained clumsy and gimpy-legged. It broke his parents' hearts to see their precious, happy-go-lucky baby boy physically disabled. The pictures taken of him showed that Little Joe could not even smile without showing marked strain on his tiny face (see photographs #3, #4, #5, and #6).

It was apparent to Dr. Faber that the child's problems arose from his traumatic birth, since physical examination of him revealed that there was a lax and unstable cervical spine. Joe's left eye was sunk towards the back of his head, and much treatment of an innovative nature was required to correct his multiple problems. The doctor decided on a course of therapy designed to overcome the patient's injurious beginnings of life.

So that he could take continuous treatment, the little boy's Aunt Beverly from the Milwaukee metropolitan area took him in as part of her family. This, even though the woman had just delivered her own newborn baby boy just two weeks before. The rest of the child's family returned to their South Dakota home, leaving Joe to be treated correctly.

As illustrated in Chapter Two, this young patient's body responded with "YES" answers to Dr. Faber's tests and selected course of treatment. Little Joe's growing body began to show signs of improvement. He underwent an intensive program of three treatments a week. His trike, which had been brought from home in Sioux Falls, was

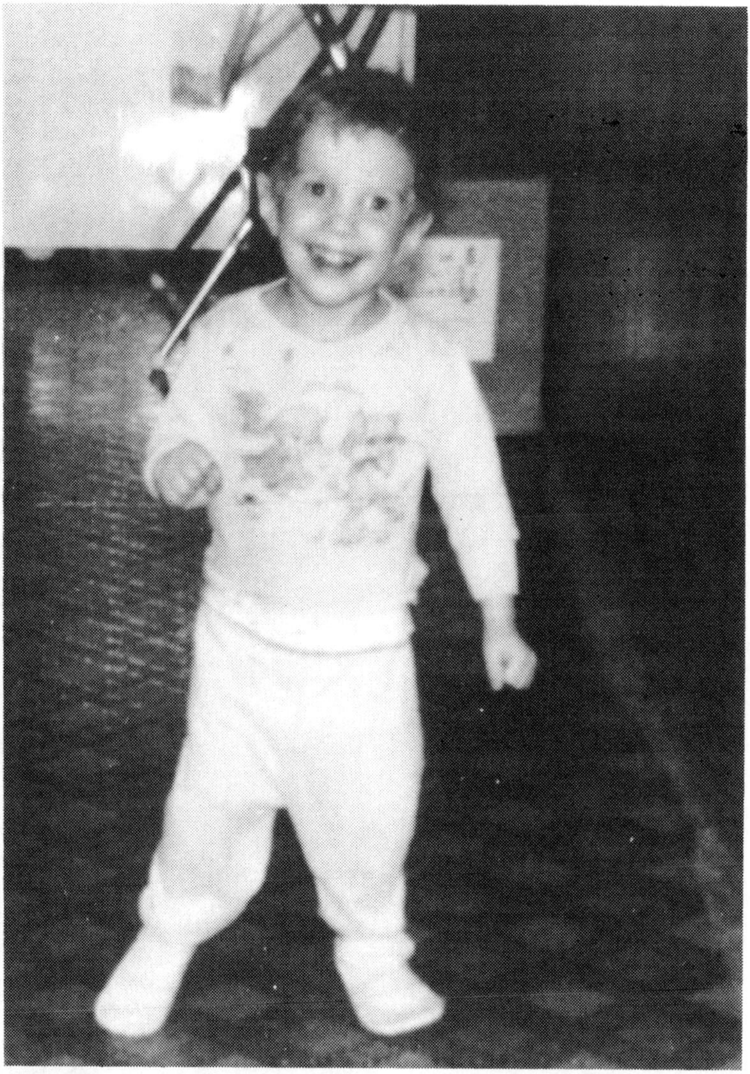

Photo #3 — As "Little Joe" grows his head tilts and eyes cross.

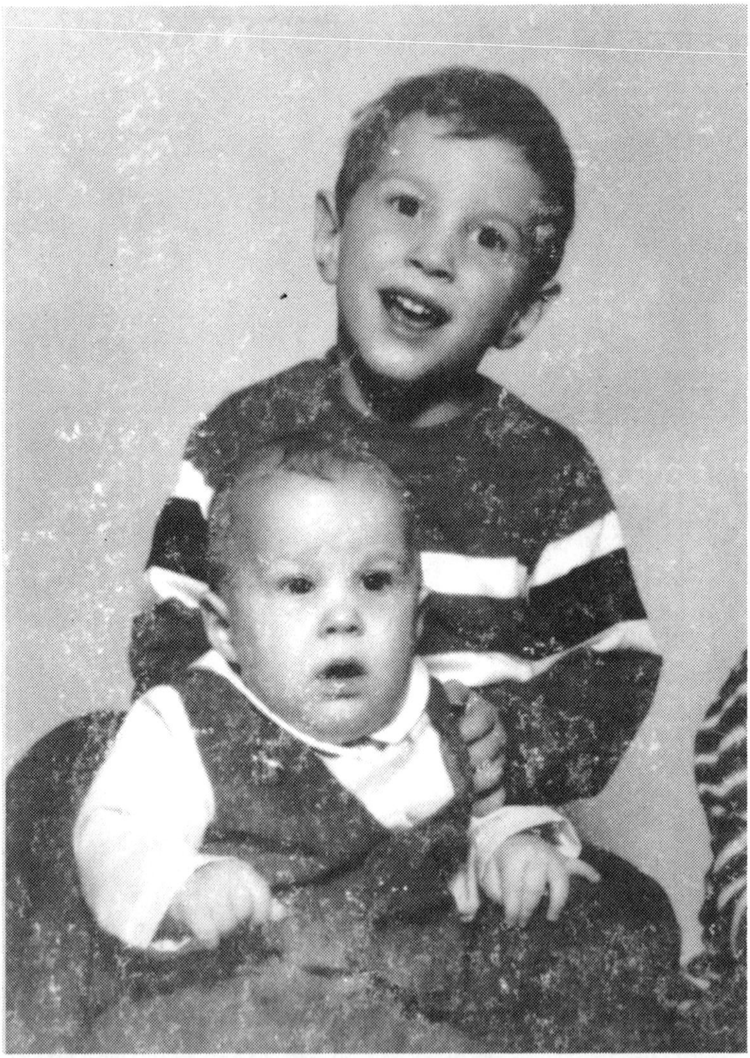

Photo #4 — As "Little Joe" grows crossed eyes and head tilt persist.

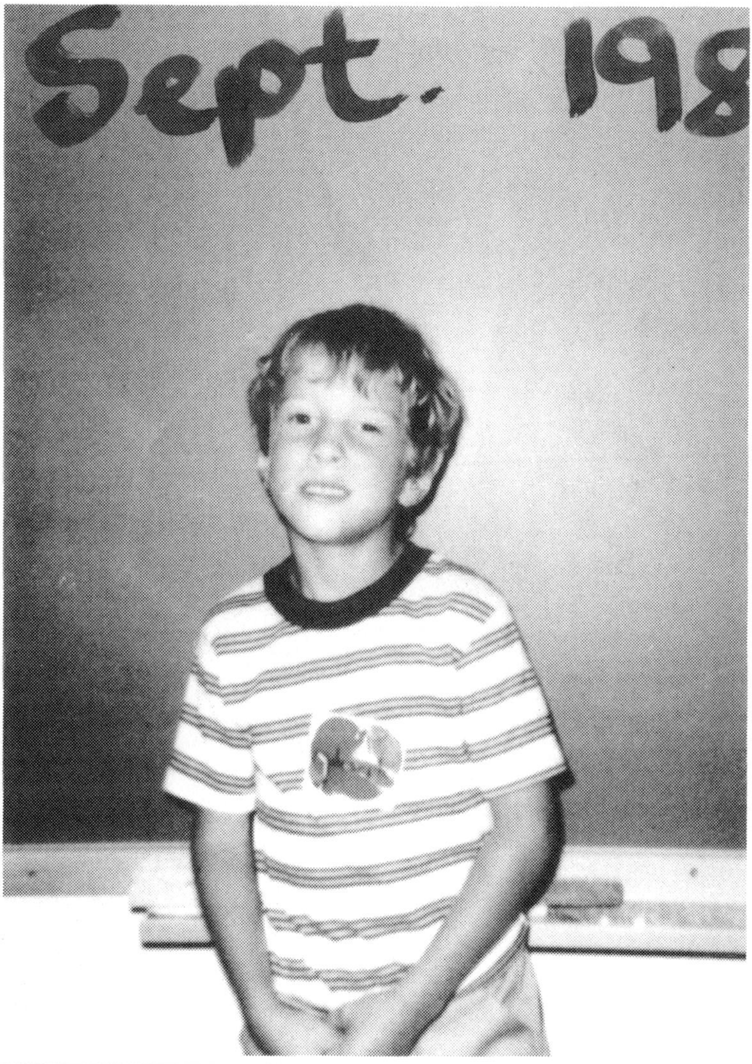

Photo #5 — Head tilt, crossed eyes and facial strain continue with "Little Joe's" growth.

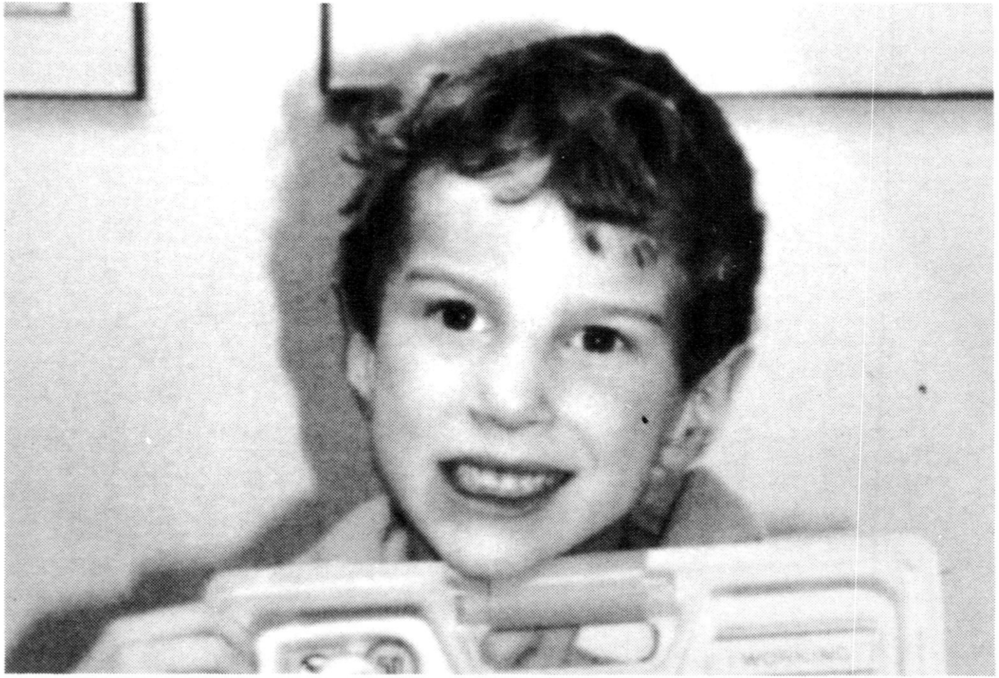

Photo #6 — Head tilt, crossed eyes and strained smile immediately prior to neural/fascial & reconstruction

mastered first by the boy. Little Joe's aunt reported that he could ride it everywhere. Then his Milwaukee swimming teacher noted that he now could swim with the best of boys his own age. Furthermore, he no longer fell repeatedly, and he held his head straight up. Doing so, prevented his neck from feeling tender and touchy. Then, his eyes stopped crossing themselves (see photograph #7).

The child is still being treated at this writing, but his relatives are highly encouraged that he will be making a nearly complete recovery from his birth trauma.

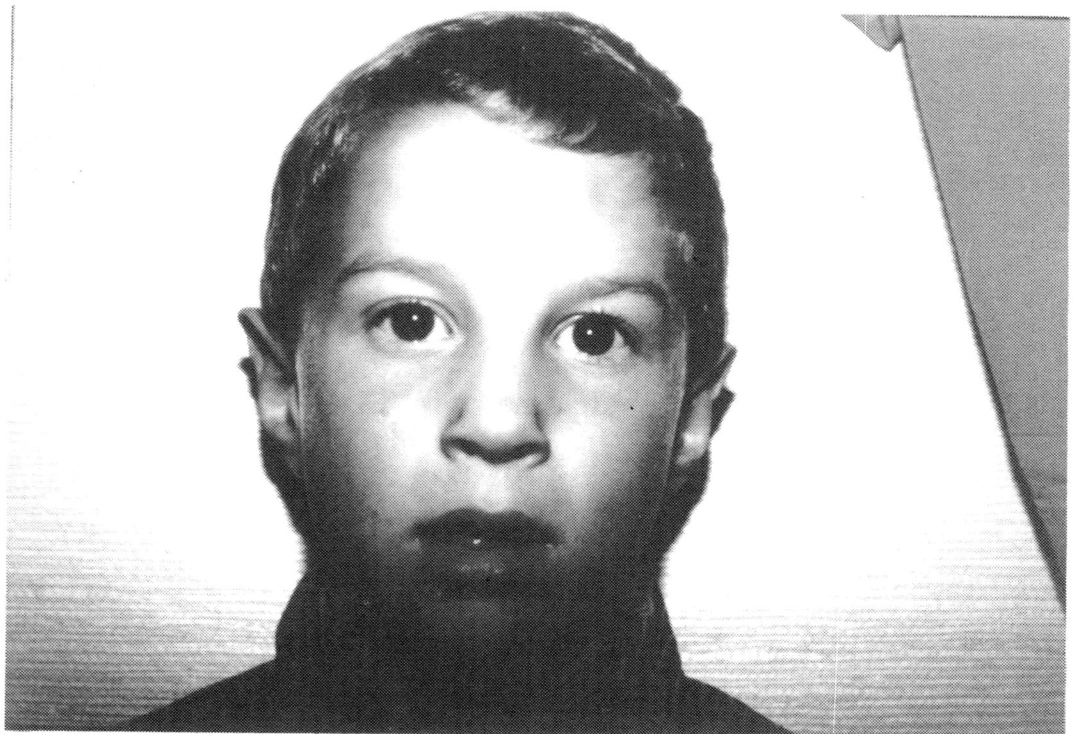

Photo #7 — After series of neural therapy "Little Joe's" eyes straighten and facial strain resolves. Head tilt was corrected with reconstruction therapy treatments.

Chapter Twelve

"HOPELESS" PATIENTS WHO ARE NOT HOPELESS ANYMORE

Biologic medicine is, above all, a recognition that detectable symptoms are but a hint that there is some underlying cause of the patient's disorder. Neural/fascial therapists who are practitioners of biological medicine realize that this underlying cause must ultimately be treated if the patient is to become healthy and whole. Predictive diagnosis seeks out these causes before they have reached the stage of clinical disease, and thus the biological method is an integral part of preventive medicine.

By means of neural/fascial therapy, patients who have been designated as "hopeless" cases become people who are not hopeless anymore. But one has the right to ask, "From where does the label 'hopeless' come? Who uses such a negative designation?" The name is given to some patients by allopathic doctors who primarily treat signs and symptoms rather than the underlying causes of disease. So long as it is dominated by the belief in specific etiology and intimately relates its treatment to the drug industry, the allopathic health care system will remain largely a disease crisis care system. This means it will remain unable to solve the bulk of our population's health problems. Today, the country's poor health is dominated not by life-threatening situations which get all the publicity, but by chronic, debilitating ones, related to lifestyle in the broadest sense. In short, these are the diseases of civilization about which we have spoken here.[1]

What follows in this chapter are just a few cases of patients who had been labelled "hopeless". Neural/fascial therapy brought them back to good repair and made them whole, functioning people once again.

Kidney Pain Removed by Neural/Fascial Therapy

An installer of hardwood floors, forty-eight-year-old Tom Foster, had visited the Milwaukee Pain Clinic to seek solutions to multiple health problems he had acquired over his life in the fast lane. One of the health-restorative procedures Dr. William Faber suggested was a deep detoxification using intravenous oxygen and oral supplementation.

About five weeks into Tom's program, a telephone call came to Dr. Faber's home at about 8:00 A.M. on Sunday from Nancy, the patient's wife. She said that her husband had been feeling awful back pain since 5:00 o'clock that same morning. Dr. Faber could hear Tom moaning from his pain in the background. Then, the patient got on the telephone and his doctor gave him three choices. He could:

1. Go to the hospital that was near to his home, about a one hour automobile ride north of Milwaukee,

2. Go to the hospital in Milwaukee of which Dr. Faber was a staff member,

3. Dr. Faber offered to travel into Milwaukee and open the pain clinic in order to consult with him.

Tom Foster took the third choice right away, and both of them traveled toward the central location. Dr. Faber recalled that Tom's X-rays during his initial medical evaluation showed a right kidney that was dropped and calcified. Also, his laboratory tests had shown considerable blood in the urine. Furthermore, a physical examination had revealed that there was kidney tenderness to touch.

In his history charts, Tom had admitted to sustaining two severe car accidents some twenty years earlier; one in which he ran into a tree at 50 miles an hour and another that occurred when his car went out of control in a field of large boulders. Tom reports that he had hit the tree so hard it tore the seat belts out of the car. He had felt back pain ever since, but it did not stop him from putting in full days as a professional flooring installer.

On that Sunday morning while lying on Dr. Faber's examining table, he couldn't do a thing to help himself except to lie still and cry out with the stabbing back pain. So, after going through with another physical examination of the patient, Dr. Faber determined that his problem arose from the dropped kidney which put a pull on the attached nerves. Assuredly, neural/fascial therapy in and around the kidney was required. It could relieve this pain.

Dr. Faber explained this to the Fosters and offered an alternative to neural/fascial therapy of being hospitalized, taking bedrest, receiving intravenous fluids, and having narcotic injections administered. Tom requested the neural/

fasical therapy. Consequently, the doctor gave his patient some superficial segmented injections first. These are small blebs of lidocaine on the skin to reset the autonomic nervous system, specifically to normalize the severe discharge of the visceral-somatic reflex mechanism. Next he injected the intercostal nerves. After carefully feeling into the kidney capsule with the hypodermic needle, there he put in some local anesthesia—lidocaine.

In just seconds after the kidney capsule was injected, the layer of stabbing pain lifted from Tom's body. He found instant pain relief. Moreover, some forty-five minutes later, Tom Foster is captured on videotape stating, "I'm feeling 100 percent better than when I came in." The mechanical aspects as well as the nerve-repairing properties of the lidocaine took out the muscle spasm and thus afforded immediate comfort against the incapacitating pain.

That Monday and for the balance of the week, Tom returned to his usual vigorous work, although he found himself needing to lie down and rest for a few hours in the evening at home. Eight days later, in for a reexamination, Tom exhibited some residual pain and spasm, for which Dr. Faber repeated the neural/fascial therapy. A repeat of the treatment was given the following week, also, even with Tom having reported that he was doing well. He had required no letup in his usual heavy work schedule. This time Dr. Faber added manual osteopathic manipulation of the man's kidney. From this last visit onward, Tom Foster has had no more problems with back pain (see photograph #8).

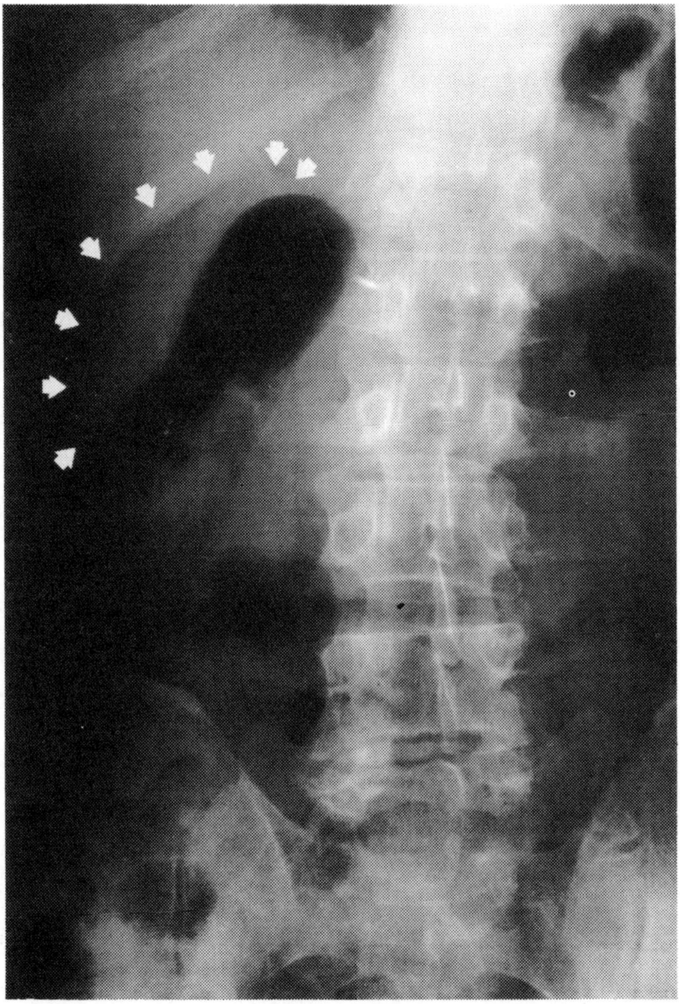

Photo #8 — X-ray with arrows showing dropped right kidney.

Restored Handwriting 25 Years After Hand Injury

Constance Endicott, at age 32, had an inability to write as required on her job as a file clerk. When she was just seven years old her hand had been injured by being slammed in a car door. The nerves and intricate muscles had been crushed. Since the problem was so well-established, the only treatment offered during her childhood was surgery on the hand tissues to bring back some semblance of control. This was not done, and she entered adulthood in an ongoing state of mental depression but accepting her disability as a fact of life.

Examined at the Milwaukee Pain Clinic by William J. Faber, D.O., Mrs. Endicott was told about neural/fascial therapy as a means of correction. She asked questions and received pertinent answers so that she understood what was involved. The doctor requested her to write her name, and it became quite apparent that she had little control over her ability to manipulate the pen and set down words intelligibly (see photograph #9).

Yet, Dr. Faber spoke confidently to her and said, "I believe the hand pain that you feel and the handwriting you seem unable to perform can be helped right away with some tiny precisely placed injections."

The patient expressed her agreement to the treatment, for she had just come from spending three weeks in the hospital for this very problem and had received no improvement under the hospital's procedures. Enthusiastically she said, "Let's do it!"

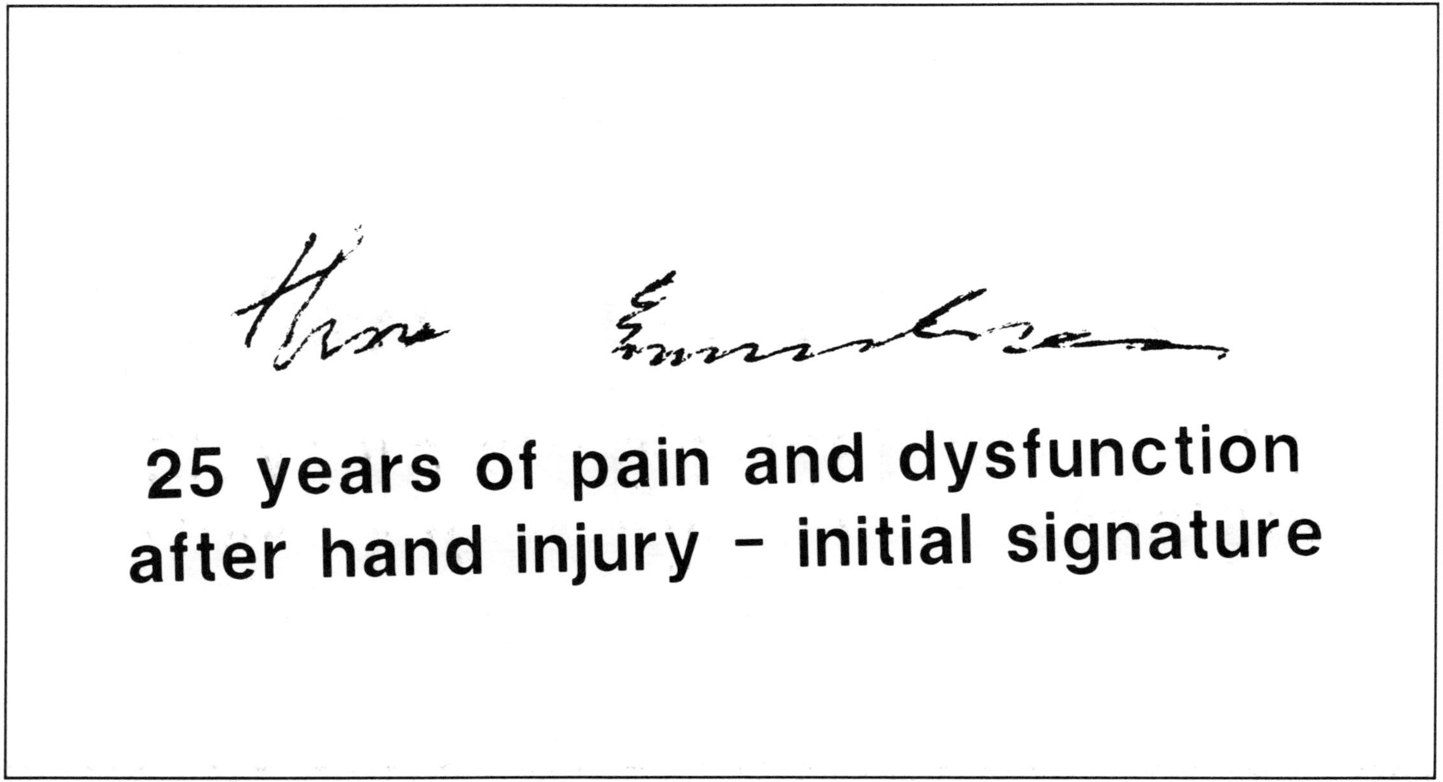

Photo #9 — Signature before neural/fascial therapy.

After freezing the hand with ethyl chloride topical anesthetic spray, Dr. Faber injected the fascia and metacarpal nerves with local anesthetic. In minutes of the injections, signs of definite improvement appeared in the hand. Twenty minutes later, Constance Endicott took up a pen and wrote her name a second time with the results of neural/ fascial therapy unmistakeable (see photograph #10). She returned to her occupation with a chance to feel more valuable in the position and a renewed zest for living.

Repair of a Knee Dysfunction

Eve Stevens brought her elderly mother, Eighty-year-old Sybil Gerry, to the Milwaukee Pain Clinic from Chicago. Mrs. Gerry had stiffness and soreness in both knees which prevented her ready mobility. After reading the patient's weight-bearing X-rays that were carried to the clinic by Mrs. Stevens, conducting a careful patient history review which had been filled out by Mrs. Gerry, and performing an orthopedic examination on the patient, Dr. Faber concluded that the knees themselves had no mechanical problems.

Odd though it may have seemed at the time, among the many areas of the doctor's examination were Mrs. Gerry's teeth, gums, and tonsils. He saw that she possessed several sites of pain where teeth had been removed years ago, and her tonsils were still intact. It occurred to him that she may have had an interference field lodged in the oral cavity (see Chapter Eleven).

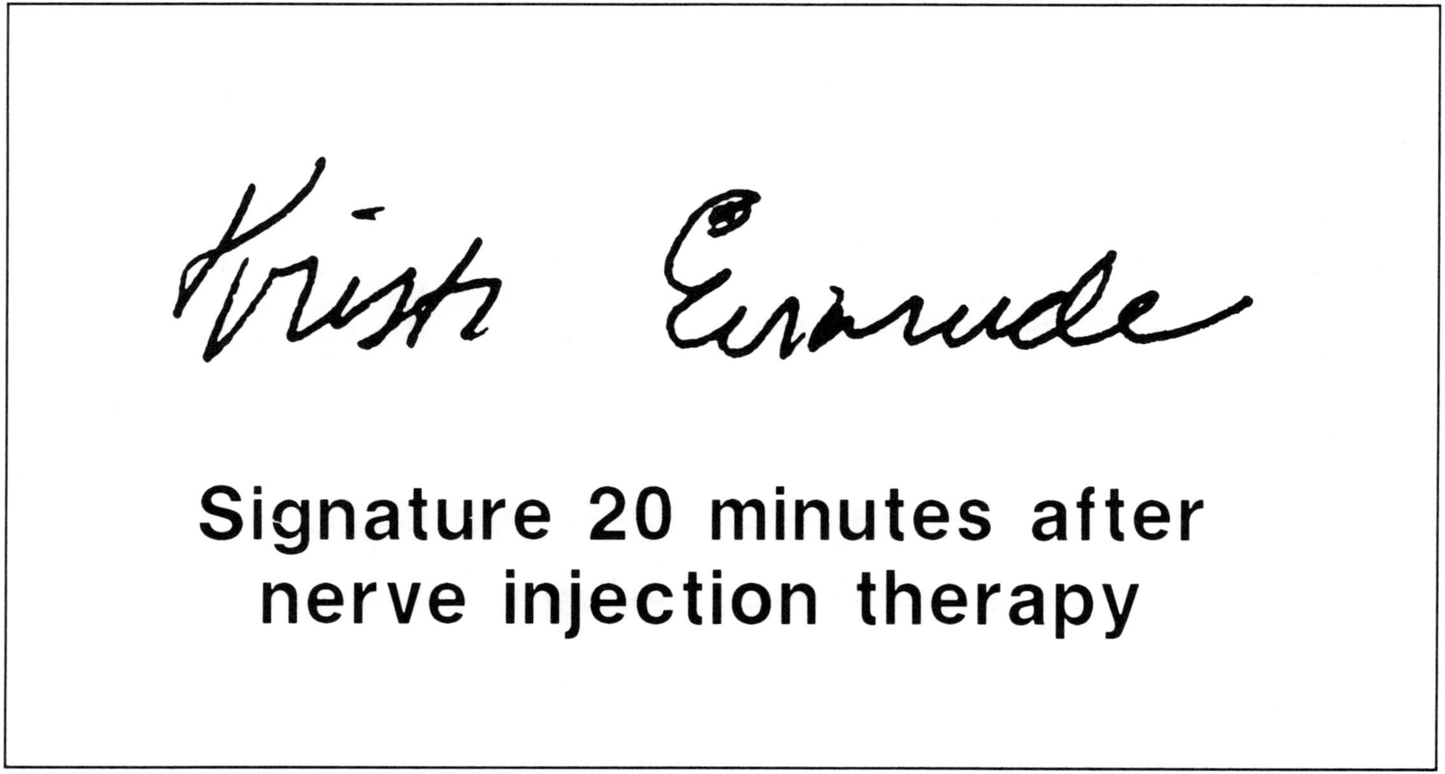

Photo #10 — Signature after neural/fascial therapy.

Dr. Faber remembered the advice of neural/fascial therapist Dietrick Klinghardt, M.D. who received international awards for his work on the healing process. Dr. Klinghardt said during the 1990 seminar of the American Academy of Biological Dentistry in Carmel Valley, California: "The knee and the tonsils appear to be on the same electrical body circuit. Always consider treating the tonsils or their scars when the patient has stiffness of the knees."

With neural/fascial treatment to Mrs. Gerry's tonsils, the patient popped off the examining table under her own power with ease. Sure enough, her tonsils were the source of difficulty for Sybil Gerry's knees. Later writing a thank you from Chicago, Eve Stevens reported that her mother had no more pain in those knees.

Pain of Amputation Relieved

Clyde Engle, 55, of Keokuk, Iowa had suffered for ten years from feeling shooting pain in his "phantom" left leg. What made it a phantom is that over a decade before, the leg had been chewed up and accidentally amputated at mid-thigh by a harvesting machine gone wild. Two weeks after his first surgical closure, the stump got infected and swelled to the point that eventually a second surgical amputation had to be carried out which took away his entire hip to the joint socket. This time, however, awakening from the operation's general anesthetic saw him sensing terrible lightning-like stabbings in the leg that no longer was there. Anytime he leaned on the hip or put some kind of pressure on his amputated side, the pains would announce themselves with vigor by stabbing him in the flesh.

The unfortunate man asked for help from Dr. William J. Faber. The treatment program that commenced included neural/fascial therapy to clear the short circuits in the patient's body. After 20 minutes of the injection procedure, it became apparent that Clyde Engle was feeling better. He could now roll and turn on the examination table. He was able to rise without feeling any of the shooting pains he had experienced daily for the prior ten years.

Having undergone only three series of neural/fascial injections to this point, he still has some residual discomfort left in the phantom limb but nothing nearly like the days of agony he suffered before (see photograph #11).

Diabetic Neuropathy Gets Instantly Removed

A diabetic individual from Madison, Wisconsin requiring over 100 units of insulin daily just to cope with living every day without symptoms of her disease. Leona Gilbert, seventy-seven years old, has a fasting blood sugar of more than 200. Even with her using Humulin RTM, the most potent and high-quality of all the insulins made by the genetic recombinant method, she still can't lower her blood sugar to near normal. As a result, the patient showed symptoms of diabetic neuropathy. She therefore traveled a distance and arrived at the Milwaukee Pain Clinic to find a way out of her misery.

"My feet feel as if they are both tingling and numb at

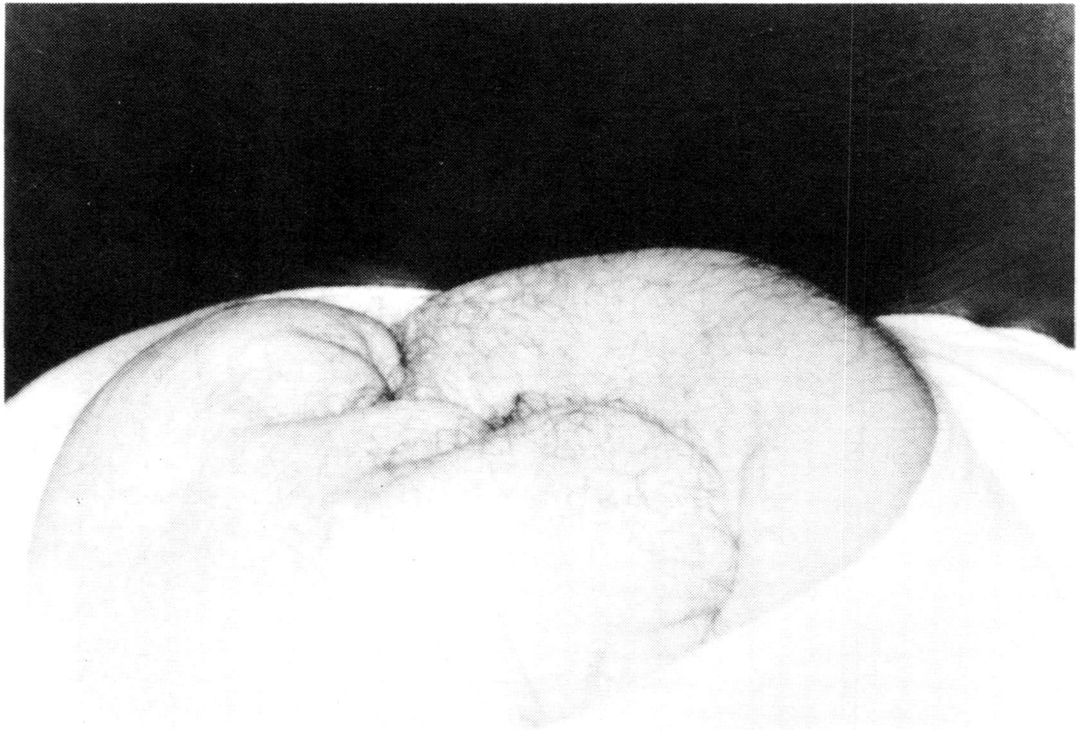

Photo #11 — Stump which caused chronic severe phantom leg pain instantly relieved with neural/fascial therapy.

the same time." The diabetic neuropathy from which she suffered, is a disease of the peripheral nerves in her legs and feet causing weakness, numbness, and sometimes an inability to tell where her feet are standing without looking. She was experiencing a lack of dorsiflexion with both feet that could not move back or up toward her shin. This crippled her gait. There were other restrictions of the muscles, blood vessels, nerves, and fascia at the top of her feet and ankles, as well.

Neural/fascial therapy solved her diabetic neuropathic problems. Dr. Faber applied space-creating treatment to the nerves and connective tissue of her feet by his injection procedure. Instantly Mrs. Gilbert felt the tingling and numbness disappear. "I can feel my feet once again; the tingling and numbness are gone," she said.

Two more treatments resolved Leona Gilbert's problem altogether, and there has been no recurrence for over a year after she received that neural/fascial therapy.

Chronic Sinus Obstruction Resolved

Gerald Warburg, eighty years old, from northeastern Ohio, arrived at the Milwaukee Pain Clinic wanting relief for his chronic back pain, which was provided by means of reconstructive therapy. During the course of his physical examination, however, Dr. Faber noticed that Mr. Warburg had a nasal deviation. When the doctor palpated his patient's nose, a lack of symmetry was revealed, and Mr. Warburg admitted to having nose breathing problems for over twenty years.

The man agreed to letting Dr. Faber attempt to correct the nose condition as well as the back problem during the same set of visits. So, carefully and with precision, neural/fascial therapy was applied in a dissecting fashion into Warburg's nose. It bled slightly, but in just minutes, the patient took a deep breath and then smiled. He said, "I can inhale real clear through my nose now. It's been forever since I could do that. I'm amazed!" He took the neural/fascial therapy for his nose one more time and that permanently restored his nasal function.

Eye Squint and Chronic Migraines Instantly Improved

Dorothy Kleiner, 67, of Green Bay, Wisconsin made her way to the Milwaukee Pain clinic after hearing Dr. Faber lecture to a health group. Dorothy relates that a friend of hers had consulted the physician and was helped. The friend recommended that Dorothy should go too.

This new patient's history revealed that she suffered pain on the left side of her face, which occurred after she slipped in the assembly plant where she works. Slipping in such a way caused Dorothy to fall to the floor, hitting the left side of her face. She consulted many neurologists and other specialists over the years and underwent all kinds of tests, screens, and X-rays. Those allopathic physicians prescribed DilantinTM, ValiumTM, ElavilTM, and all sorts of pain medications such as Tylenol #4TM, DarvonTM, Fiorinal #3TM, VicodinTM, and others. After a while, Dorothy noticed that the pills made her sick and reduced her energy. Such drug side effects were upsetting her terribly.

Dr. Faber's examination revealed that the patient had irritated cranial and facial nerves which caused increased muscular tensions of the tiny muscles which controlled the eye lids. The result was a right eye that appeared to be smaller than the left one (see photograph # 12). The doctor explained to Dorothy that he believed she was an ideal candidate for instant pain relief of her chronic migraine pain.

The patient immediately agreed to the neural/fascial injections to her head and face. Dr. Faber used the German neural therapy technique with his own innovations (neural/fascial therapy) to the nerves of the affected temporal, facial, and occipital nerves. In seconds, he could see the desired results had taken place, and he took a photograph (see photograph #13). Dorothy felt immediately that her pain was gone for the first time in so many years. For the patient, the relief was a miracle. For Dr. Faber, it was routine.

Upon his advice, she returned in a week for another series of injections. Dorothy was overjoyed that she felt so much improvement. The chronic facial and head migraine were much diminished but not entirely gone, and eliminating it altogether was Dr. Faber's goal. He applied the treatment again as determined by his examination. Her improvement continued until after a total of ten injection sessions, her penetrating and torturous migraines were over for good.

Not only did she have no more discomfort, but Dorothy's energy came back as if she was a youngster. Previous to

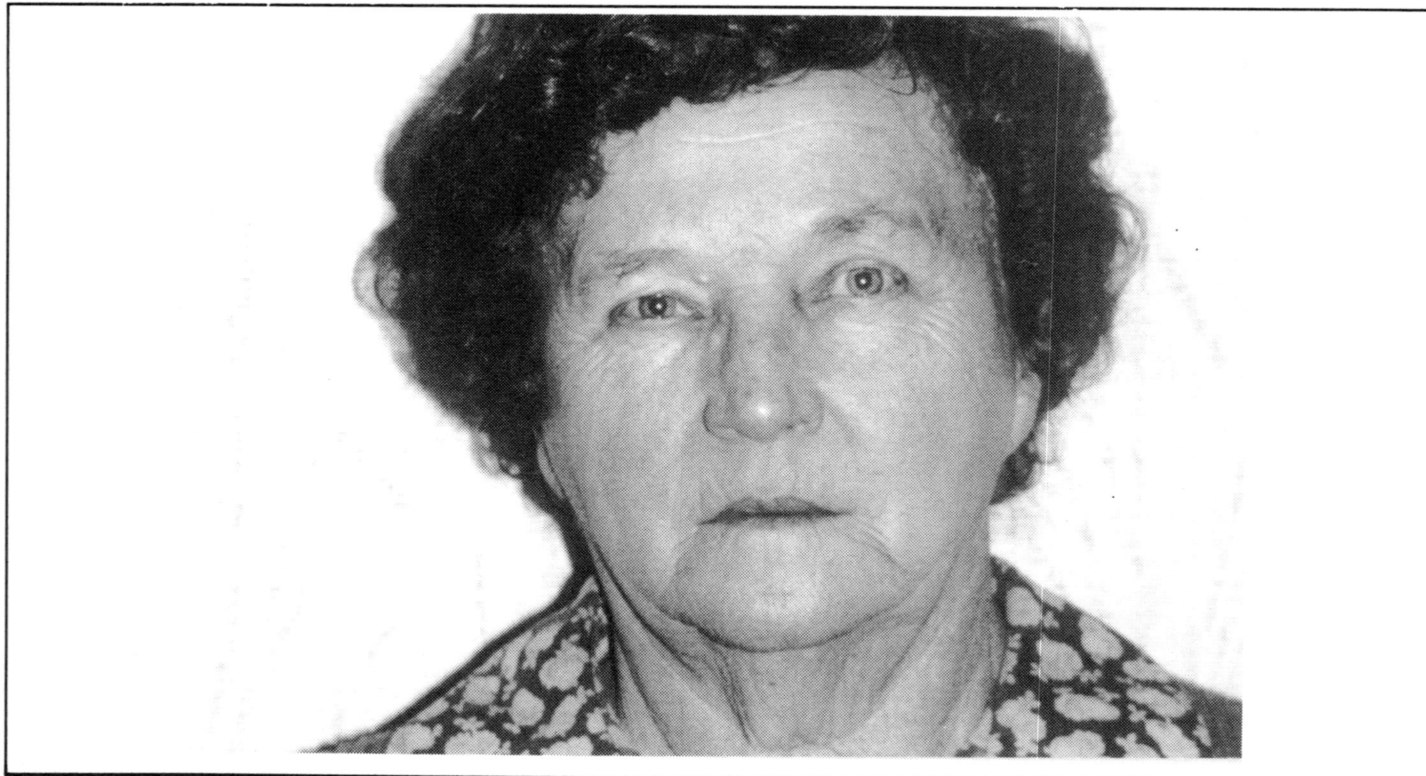

Photo #12 — D.K. suffered migraines after striking her head 20 years ago. Note eyes prior to neural/fascial therapy.

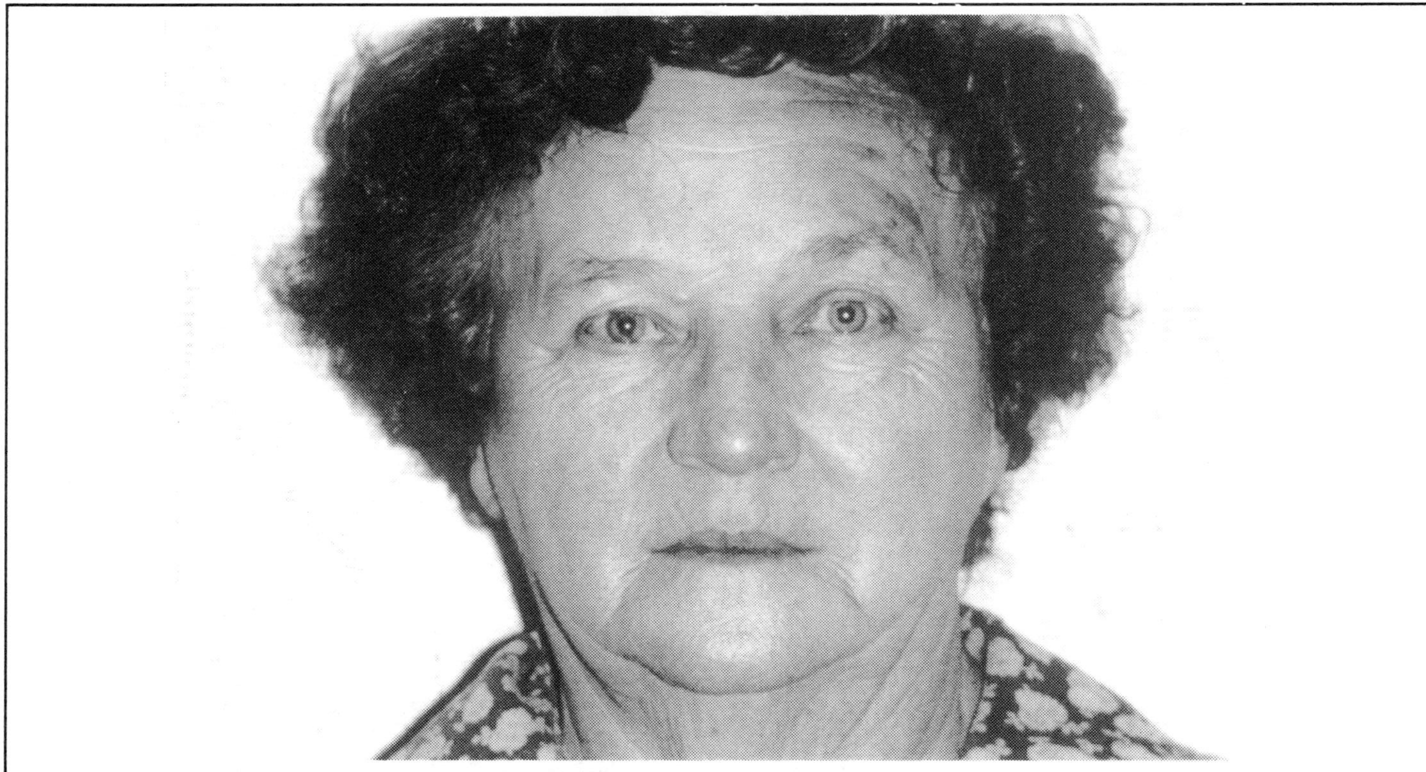

Photo #13 — D.K. immediately after neural/fascial treatment. Note change of eyes.

treatment she could not gather strength enough even to mow her own lawn or shovel snow off her driveway. Now Dorothy Kleiner could accomplish those individual tasks and had energy to spare.

It has been seven months since the woman's head pain has been resolved. For her there has been no recurrences and none are expected.

Contractures of the Hands Instantly Improved

As stated earlier, loss of range of motion can be due to calcifications and adhesions of tissue. This occurred in the case of Charles Klone of Moline, Illinois. Charlie suffered from severe polio for 45 years which so weakened his legs that he required the use of heavy steel braces in order to walk without crutches. Reconstructive therapy (see Pain, Pain Go Away) rebuilt his ankles, knees, back and hips to the extent that his walking ability dramatically improved.

Being a never-say-die kind of person, Charlie decided he was going to seek help from Dr. Faber for contractures of his hands as well. Interestingly, Charlie practiced with a therapeutic technique himself. He had quite a following as a reflexologist and used his fingers constantly to give comfort to the feet and bodies of others. For himself, however, he could not administer reflexology. (Reflexology is the science of manipulating the hands and feet of somebody else in order to send nerve impulses to their body organs and structures so as to stimulate them to function correctly.) Charlie's fingers maintained themselves in a state of spasm and contracture, and the subsequent pain that goes with this condition is immense. His hand contractions, tendon spasms, and deformities were quite apparent (see photograph #14).

Dr. Faber's examination of Charles Klone's hands revealed, among other abnormalities, a loss of flexion at the wrist. The doctor believed that the loss of motion came from calcification developing in the extensor tendon sheaths. Upon applications of neural/fascial therapeutic injections an immediate and permanent increase of wrist motion was obtained for this man (see photograph #15).

Traumatic Vertigo Resolved with Neural/Fascial Therapy

Fifty-six-year-old Raymond Price suffered from severe spinning dizziness even from merely turning over in bed. He also had awful headaches and visited the Milwaukee Pain Clinic in order to find some relief from both sets of symptoms. Raymond connected his headaches to an incident occurring two years before when he rose from a squatting position and struck his head on an overhanging shelf. The blow was so severe that it gave his neck vertebrae a compression fracture. Subsequent to the injury, a neurosurgeon performed a fusion operation of the neck, taking bone chips out of the patient's hip. After taking a few months off to recuperate from the surgery and hospitalization, Raymond was able to return to his usual occupation of building houses. Still, with all that he had gone trough, his headaches remained.

Then, two months before he found his way to the

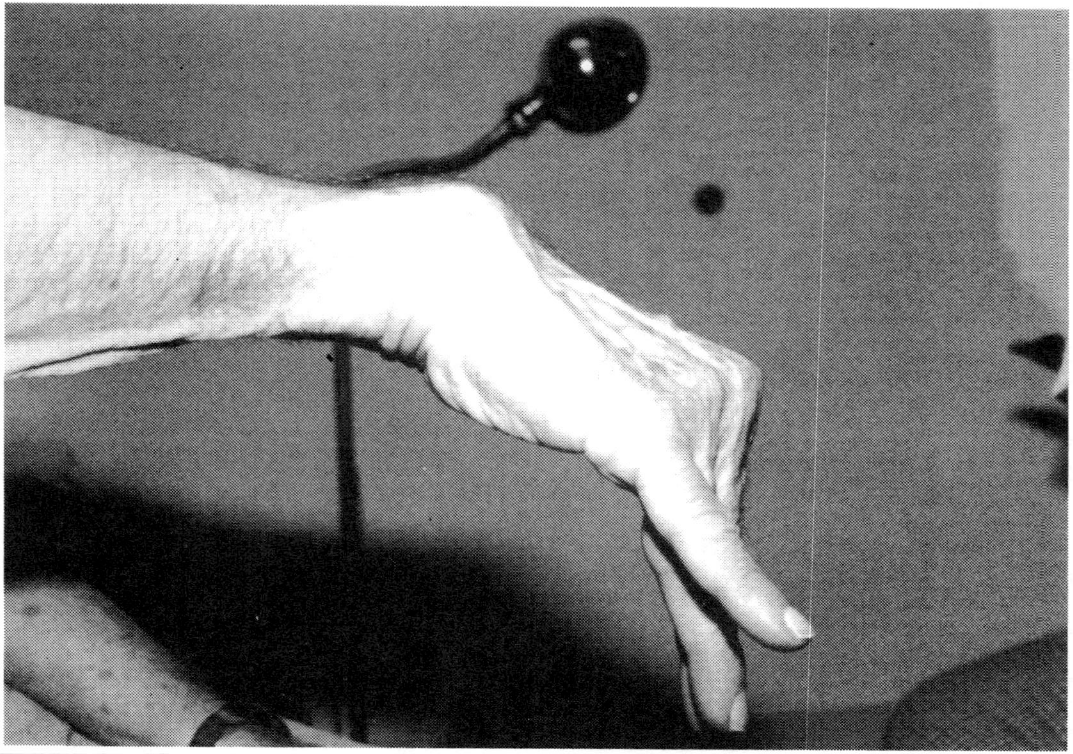

Photo #14 — Charles K. maximum flexion of wrist.

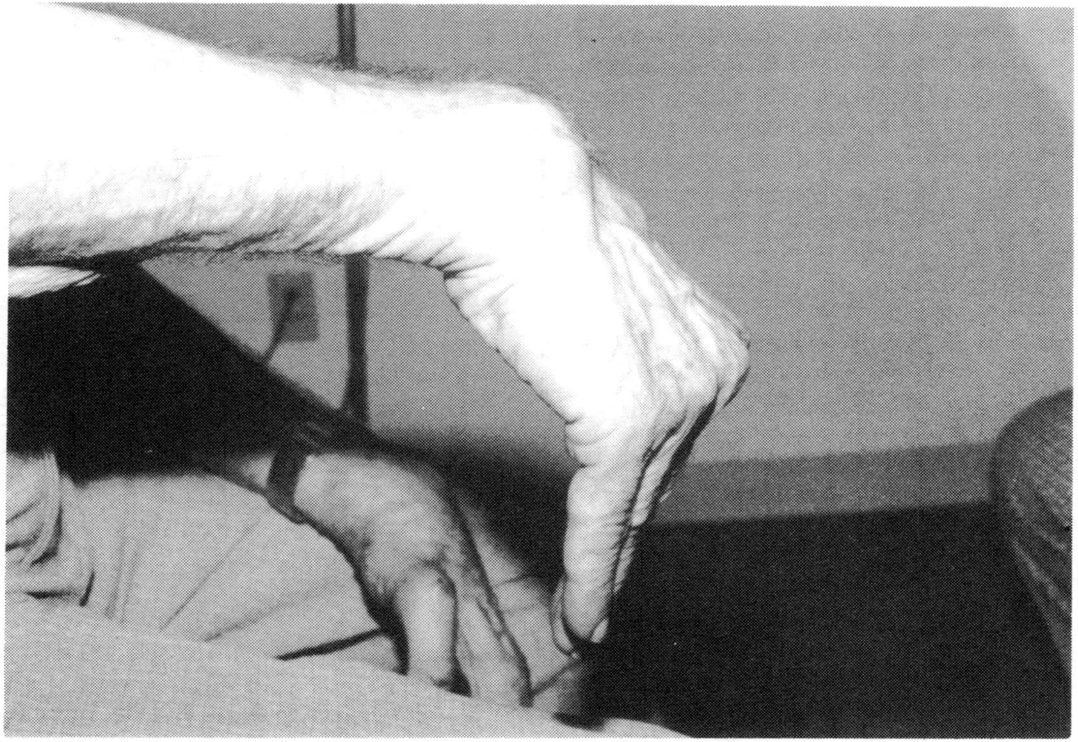

Photo #15 — Charles K. maximum wrist flexion immediately after neural/fascial therapy.

Milwaukee Pain Clinic, the dizziness began for him. It was more than the tough builder could handle, and Dr. Faber's treatment program was his last best hope. Raymond agreed to suggestions made by the physician. Reconstructive therapy to rebuild the man's torn and compressed neck ligaments and bone was applied in a repeated series of injections. From a long distance away in central Wisconsin, the patient was driven to the clinic by a relative. Nevertheless, he was happy to make the trip and find comfort. And comfort did come to him, for the next week he gratefully reported, "My headache is 90 percent better, but there is no change in my feeling of dizziness." In fact, he reported having vertigo just getting on the examination table at that second consultation.

It was then that Dr. Faber decided to add neural/fascial therapy to his armamentarium of treatment for this man. He administered the crown and occipital nerve techniques which he routinely teaches to other physicians during the course of their preceptorships with him. Requesting that Raymond test the efficacy of the injection techniques just applied, Dr. Faber had the patient get up and down repeatedly. Sure enough, the dizziness was gone—the same dizziness the patient had been experiencing just minutes before.

At this time—even as we are going to press—Raymond Price is still receiving his treatments. Dr. Faber predicts that the builder will have total recovery after the full and necessary series of neural/fascial injections are done.

Chapter Thirteen

ANSWERS TO QUESTIONS ABOUT NEURAL/FASCIAL THERAPY

If neural/fascial therapy is so good and effective, why aren't the big medical centers and many more doctors doing it?

More physicians are learning how to give the treatment. To now, however, only about 5,000 doctors around the world know the methods for administering it—an insufficient number. The greatest reason there are not more is because the pharmaceutical industry largely runs the practice of allopathic medicine in most industrialized nations. The local anesthetics applied in neural/fascial therapy are lidocaine, procaine, and some others. These have come off patent years ago so that using them does not generate hugh profits for the pharmaceutical industry. Without a good financial return from promoting these anesthetics, no drug company is prepared to invest advertising money or door-to-door detailing of them to clinics, hospitals, and doctors' offices. Only the enthusiasm of pioneering physicians using neural/fascial therapy keeps it alive and available.

What is the frequency of administration of neural/fascial therapy for achieving permanent resolution of a health problem?

The health problem's magnitude is the primary factor so that the series of required injections vary from one to twenty. Being both diagnostic and therapeutic, value is found in giving the treatment at any opportunity. Neural/fascial therapy is expected to work in a step-wise improvement pattern with each additional application.

How quickly can an individual go through a usual neural/fascial therapy program and receive maximum results?

Treatment of patients daily for two weeks offers the maximum effect. There is a quantum leap in pain reduction this way. Function improves, too, along with endurance and energy. People traveling hundreds of miles will probably arrive weekly and stay overnight so that treatments can be received back to back. They repeat this weekly visitation or two week until maximum permanent benefit is obtained.

What side effects are there with neural/fascial therapy?

Even with the injection of up to 200 cubic centimeters of anesthetic solution, there have been no significant adverse side effects. It's one of the safer forms of treatment. Yet the knowledge, training and skill of an individual neural/fascial therapist is a factor. Bruising with its attendant soreness and skin discoloration is the most common irritation that might accompany the treatment. Or, a patient could have prolonged numbness or soreness after a series of neural/fascial injections, but these go away relatively quickly.

Hidden infections and other illnesses may become apparent due to the stimulation and "opening up" effects of neural-fascial therapy. Necessary to be mentioned is that it's contraindicated to give the therapy to a patient who is on cortisone because this drug blocks the human body's neural- and tissue-healing pathways.

Upon visiting a neural/fascial therapist for the first time, should I bring along my medical reports and X-ray films?

Yes, present the doctor with any records that will help in the diagnosis and treatment program. Every bit as important as these is for you to present a written history of your past injuries, infections, operations, dental work, drug treatments, reactions, and other traumatic events. Assist your doctor in returning to the earliest causes of your health problems.

What is the cost of a course of neural/fascial treatment?

Fees are based on the standard regional anesthesia fee listings. To learn of charges by the individual doctor whom you are consulting, telephone or write that doctor for exact information.

Are results with neural/fascial therapy guaranteed?

No. But often it does work when all other therapies have failed. Only death, taxes and governmental incompetency in life are guaranteed.

Is neural/fascial therapy covered by health insurance?

The quality of the particular insurance policy you carry will determine this answer. Quality coverage pays for the injection of nerves, which this treatment does. As we mentioned earlier in the book, the most costly treatment is that particular therapy which does not work. Still, the individual clinic at which you are consulting will probably have the most accurate answer to this valid question.

Does this book describe all of the conditions for which neural/fascial therapy has usefulness?

No. Although the case histories given are true—about real patients and their physicians—they are only representative.

What conditions are not helped by neural/fascial therapy?

Infections, cancer, arteriosclerosis, angina pectoris, schizophrenia, Parkinson's disease, senile dementia, and some other metabolic conditions are not cured or improved by the application of neural/fascial therapy. Neural/fascial therapy may be of value in conjuction with other treatments.

Chapter Fourteen

Actual Patient Case Histories

While this book was being written it was discovered that medical society guidelines prohibiting patient names disclosure have been lifting. This book has been delayed in its release date to compile the following actual case histories. Since these people are kind enough to share their stories and communicate it with others searching for relief it requested the following guidelines be used.

1. Always be courteous. These people are answering questions to help you.

2. Ask if you are calling at an acceptable time. If you ask them to call you back, allow them to call collect.

3. If you write, always include a stamped self addressed envelope for your response.

4. Thank the person for sharing their time and experiences with you.

The authors extend their sincerest gratitudes to following people for allowing others in suffering to contact them so that they may start on their healing path. Life is often tough, it's sure a help when someone farther down the road gives a report. These persons have consented on their own free will without any compensation to expose their life stories. We salute their noble kindness to help strangers not finding relief of their pain.

Due to the nature of the problems some patients were given neural-fascial and reconstruction therapy concurrently. An occasional patient may have only been given neural-fascial or reconstruction therapy.

These people have given us their written permission according to medical society rules. Their signatures are in our files.

SEVERE SCOLIOSIS AND BACK PAIN

Anne Lion Niemi
Alpine Residence, Gulf Road
Roscoe, New York 12776
Tel: 607-498-5263

Pain in lower back started about 3 1/2 to 4 years ago. Went to a Dr. Bach in Rhinebeck, NY but Dr. would not treat her with the needles.

Patient states since starting treatments with Dr. Faber she feels stronger and firmer. Patient had previously been treated for yeast infection in the Rhinebeck Clinic. Patient's abdomen has shifted to the side. Patient has had problem with eyes and after the IV treatments at Clinic, her eyes are somewhat improved.

Patient is having less pain in the back than when she first visited the Clinic. Patient states pain starts in back and goes into the front abdomen. She is being helped by injections. Anyone may call her.

You may publish story.

Anne Lion Niemi

SEVERE KNEE DEGENERATION

Luella McEvoy
4215 N. 10th St.
Milwaukee, WI 53102
Te: 1-462-2567

I have had pain in my right knee and could hardly walk.

I attended a lecture that Dr. Faber gave and I decided to call the Milwaukee Pain Clinic for an appointment.

I started taking the injection therapy from Dr. Faber and

(Turn to Page 213 before contacting these people.)

I found I have no pain now. I have greater strength and am able to work so much better and my knees feel so much firmer.

I would be glad to talk to anyone that calls me and tell them how pleased I am with the treatment at Milwaukee Pain Clinic.

You may publish my story.

Luella McEvoy

RINGING OF EARS, NECK AND BACK PAIN RESOLVED

David Speer
2305 8th St.
Silvis, IL 61282
Tel: 706-792-8180

I had my first chiropractic visits in 1980 and about every 6 months - later on I moved to Arizona where I had some back injury. I had a slipped disc and began going to a chiropractor out in Arizona about 3 times a week for 2 years. During that time I had constant headaches and back aches. The manipulations did not hold. I moved back to Illinois where I met Dr. Odvarko and she began a detoxification program and stretching exercises. I went once a week for adjustments. After seeing her for 1 year, Dr. Odvarko sent me to Milwaukee Pain Clinic to see Dr. Faber. At the time I was seeing Dr. Odvarko, I had ringing in my ear which would not go away.

I came to Dr. Faber and he had me X-rayed. The X-rays showed I had some head trauma. Dr. Faber started injection into my back and it is slowly strengthening my back.

Dr. Faber then began to work on the ringing in my ears. Dr. Faber injected my ear, my ear popped and the ringing is entirely gone.

(Turn to Page 213 before contacting these people.)

When I first came to Milwaukee Pain Clinic I had really bad pain. After Dr. Faber's treatment the pain is so much better.

If it was not for the treatments I received at the Milwaukee Pain Clinic I would probably be dead by now.

I would be very happy to discuss these treatments with anyone that calls me.

You may publish my story.

David Speer

CRIPPLING PAIN OF THE FEET INSTANTLY RESOLVED

Sharon Monnin
906 N. Browns Lake Rd.
Burlington, WI
Te: 414-534-5384

Sometime in September or October I came to the Milwaukee Pain Clinic and had blood tests and thyroid tests done. It was found my immune system was really out of whack. What brought me to Pain Clinic was severe crippling pain in the bottom of my feet. I couldn't walk or bend either foot. I hobbled around for many weeks and things didn't get better.

When I came to the Clinic (on my second visit) I had the results of my blood test and Dr. Faber suggested a treatment for my feet. He injected my head that day, with the treatment taking 15 to 20 minutes. I got up off the table, and there was absolutely no pain. I walked for the first time normally, after at least 6 weeks of constant pain. I have had no further treatment for the pain in the last 2 years. The pain was so severe I couldn't tell if it was bone pain or muscular pain.

(Turn to Page 213 before contacting these people.)

I will gladly talk to anyone that will call me. I honestly thought I was a cripple for life.

You may publish my story.

Sharon Monnin

SEVERE DISC DISEASE THROUGHOUT THE ENTIRE SPINE

Patricia Lang
2164 Bear Creek Rd.
Stevens Point, WI 54481
Tel: 715-344-3409

I had a pain in my back all the time. I was very apprehensive when I came to the Milwaukee Pain Clinic to see Dr. Faber, and I wondered if it was going to work. I had read the book Pain, Pain, Go Away and wondered what the treatment was about.

After the first treatment, I felt the treatment was going to work because I immediately got some relief.

Whatever happened since then, as far as the treatments are concerned, are great because my back is so much better. It is 100% better.

I would be happy to talk to anyone that would call me about how happy I am with my results at Milwaukee Pain Clinic.

You may publish my story.

Patricia Lang

(Turn to Page 213 before contacting these people.)

CHRONIC HEADACHES AND UNRELIEVED BACK PAIN

Glorianne Pawlak
4061 Reforestation Rd.
Green Bay, WI 54313
414-434-2428

When I first came to Milwaukee Pain Clinic, I had pain in my lower back. I had spondylosis and spondylolisthesis and severe headaches. I had headaches for years. I read the book by Dr. Faber called Pain, Pain Go Away. I read the book and then I heard Dr. Faber speak in Green Bay. What he said made good sense to me.

Since I started treatment at Milwaukee Pain Clinic I feel so much better. My headaches are so much better and my back is getting better all the time.

I am so happy I came to the Milwaukee Pain Clinic and very happy with my progress.

I would gladly talk to anyone that calls me about how much better I feel since the treatments.

You may publish my story.

Glorianne Pawlak

HIDDEN JAW PROBLEM & CHRONIC BACK & KNEE ARTHRITIS

Elva Boyd
10119 221st Ave. N. W.
Elk River, Minn 55330
Tel: 612-441-4780

When I first went to the Milwaukee Pain Clinic I had pain in my back and left knee. Dr. Faber thought I had an

(Turn to Page 213 before contacting these people.)

infection in both of my jaws and I went to my own dentist and an orthodontist and another dentist that does root canals. They argued there was nothing wrong. It is impossible because the root was dead because of the root canals. So I just gave up. I had X-rays from my regular dentist four years in a row. The dentist could not find anything wrong.

Dr. Faber ordered X-rays of my whole jaw and found the infection in my jaws. Dr. Faber referred me to Dr. Spaeth and he did surgery in 4 areas - when the dentist went into the upper gums he had to go into the sinus area on both sides. There was a lot of infection on both sides. This was in the middle of December when I had surgery on my gums - and by the middle of January I noticed the pain in my head was gone. I find I can think better and concentrate better. The last few weeks I can think clearly. The pain in my mouth is gone. The fogginess is gone.

I started treatment at Milwaukee Pain Clinic on my back and knees and I see an improvement.

I will gladly discuss my treatment by Dr. Faber at Milwaukee Pain Clinic and I can highly recommend him.

You may publish my story.

Elva E. Boyd

TERRIBLE STOMACH, NECK AND BACK PAINS OF MANY YEARS RESOLVED

Joe Bach
14600 Woodland Dr.
New Berlin, WI 53151
Tel: 1-786-4566

I came to Milwaukee Pain Clinic because of terrible digestive problems along with stomach problems. I had pain in my neck and back and radiating down my legs.

(Turn to Page 213 before contacting these people.)

After Dr. Faber started the injections, I noticed immediate relief in the back and neck. I continued the treatment and my back and neck are so much better. My digestive problems have improved so much. My back was so uncomfortable.

I am now feeling so much better. I would be glad to discuss my treatments at the Milwaukee Pain Clinic. It made me feel wonderful. I feel more peaceful.

You may publish my story.

Joe Bach

SEVERE NECK PAIN FROM DEGENERATIVE DISCS

Rosina Hahn
W 1628 Hy O
Oconomowoc, WI 53066
414-474-4398

At least 2 years ago my neck started having pain and I could not turn my head from side to side, had trouble sitting, could hardly drive my car and I could not do any of my housework. My neck just had so much pain.

I heard Dr. Faber from the Milwaukee Pain Clinic on the radio and I decided to come to see him.

Dr. Faber started injecting my neck and the injections certainly did so much good. My neck now feels fine.

My feet started to hurt several years ago and I could hardly walk. I was so unsteady all the time. At the Milwaukee Pain Clinic Dr. Faber started injections on my feet and after the first treatment I felt more stability. My feet now feel wonderful.

I will be glad to tell anyone about the help I received at

(Turn to Page 213 before contacting these people.)

the Milwaukee Pain Clinic.

You may publish my story and I hope you do.

Rosina M. Hahn

CHRONIC PAIN ON LEFT SIDE & HEADACHES INSTANTLY RESOLVED

Dorothy Rubitsky
Rt 1 603 W. Main
Palmyra, WI 53156
414-495-2814

I have had pain on my whole left side from my neck down. The pain was in my hip, back, and knee.

I heard Dr. Faber on the radio talking about Reconstructive Therapy and I decided to call him to see if he could help me. I had been to so many doctors over the years with no help. Since I have been coming to Milwaukee Pain Clinic, my neck and shoulder feel so much better than it has in years and with only 2 treatments.

I will continue to have treatments on my back and hip at Milwaukee Pain Clinic because I am confident that the injection therapy works.

I will gladly talk to anyone about the treatments at Milwaukee Pain Clinic. The people at the Pain Clinic are so friendly. I know Dr. Faber will be able to help the hip problem.

You may publish my story.

Dorothy Rubitsky

(Turn to Page 213 before contacting these people.)

NUMBNESS OF FINGERS FROM NECK INSTABILITY

Dudley McClain
290 Normandy Ln.
Grayslake, IL 60030
Tel: 708-223-0829

I had a lot of numbness in my fingers since last February and this was a very annoying feeling and I was afraid my fingers were going to get worse.

My chiropractor recommended I see Dr. Faber at the Milwaukee Pain Clinic. I came in, talked to Dr. Faber, and I received treatment the first time. I noticed immediate relief and the numbness started to go away. After I continued the treatment the numbness has almost disappeared.

I am very satisfied with all my treatments at the Milwaukee Pain Clinic and with the injections Dr. Faber gave me.

I will definitely talk to anyone that calls me.

You may publish my story.

Dudley McClain

SPONDYLOLISTHESIS CAUSING SEVERE BACK PAIN AND DISABILITY

Ethel Klug
38388 Mapleton Rd.
Oconomowoc, WI 53066
Tel: 414-474-7092

Since the birth of my third child, 48 years ago I have had back problems. I went to several different doctors and was diagnosed as having Spondylolisthesis. I went to a Neurologist and he suggested I have surgery. I then went to a

(Turn to Page 213 before contacting these people.)

chiropractor but the treatment, were too hard and was rough for me to take so I stopped going.

I heard Dr. Faber on the radio and I decided to come and see him to see if he could help my terrible pain.

Dr. Faber started injecting my back and I noticed relief right away. Since taking treatments from Dr. Faber my back is so much stronger and I do not have to wear the elastic support belt. I do not have to use a pillow to support my back any longer. My back feels terrific and I am so happy with my treatment at the Milwaukee Pain Clinic.

I would be glad to discuss the great results I received at the Milwaukee Pain Clinic.

You may publish my story.

Ethel Klug

CHRONIC LOW BACK PAIN

Janet Kaufman
560 Forrest Road
Cookeville, TN 38501
615-528-6979

National Chronic Pain
Outreach Association, Inc.
7979 Old Georgetown Road, Suite 100
Bethesda, MD 20814-2429

To Whom It May Concern:

My subscription runs out with this issue, and the timing seems to be perfect! I have just returned from the Milwaukee Pain Clinic (Dr. William Faber) where I received the beginning of my Proliferative or Reconstruction Therapy (6 out of

(Turn to Page 213 before contacting these people.)

18 or 30 treatments), and for the first time in two years, I can sit and walk upright for more than 1/2 hour without excruciating pain.

I learned of this treatment after reading Dr. Faber's book, Pain, Pain Go Away, and knew in my heart that this was probably for me. I injured my back after a fall two years ago, and have not had a satisfactory (to me) diagnosis or prognosis since. Dr. Faber diagnosed me as having a lumbar ligament involvement.

His therapy is not new (it's been around since the 30's, I believe), and is just beginning to gain notoriety. I met patients in his waiting room that have come back from total disability to walking around with smiles on their faces. One patient I spoke with says she is 70% better and expects in the next few visits to reach 100%. That is my goal!

Reconstruction Therapy is used to treat damaged, stretched or torn ligaments, problems with tendons and joints. (I rejected it at first, because I believed my problem was nerve/disk related. They told me that oftentimes ligaments are involved, if not directly in the actual nerve pain, then indirectly—a strengthened ligament can keep a disc in place. And even a stretched or torn ligament can cause nerves that will always hurt.)

Once the diagnosis is made, the problem area is injected with a natural irritant solution (e.g. sodium chloride, and lidocaine) to cause a controlled inflammation. The body is then stimulated to heal—laying down new tissue, rebuilding torn ligaments, shoring up stretched ones. (There's more, particularly concerning knees, arthritis, etc. but you'll have to get that from the book.)

The therapy works with your body's own healing process,

(Turn to Page 213 before contacting these people.)

so it is essential that your nutritional level and immune system are both exceptional. If not, they do testing and adjust whatever needs adjustment. The therapy is uncomfortable (what injections aren't?), but the outcome is permanent... and it is effective in 88-92% of the patients on whom it is performed.

READ THE BOOK! It's definitely worth looking into. The Milwaukee Pain Clinic is located at 6529 Fond du Lac Avenue, Milwaukee, WI 53218, and their phone number is 414-464-PAIN.

With hope that this will help others, I am

Sincerely yours,

Janet Kaufman

CHRONIC LOW BACK PAIN FROM HYPERMOBILITY SYNDROME

NEWSPAPER ARTICLE

THE BUDGET - Wednesday, October 24, 1990 - Page 21

To all those out there who have been inquiring and/or suffering from chronic joint pain, TMJ, migraines, Carpal Tunnel, arthritis, hip and knee pain and all other joint related diseases - there is an alternative to surgery and drugs. Read all about it in the new book Pain, Pain Go Away, by Dr. Wm. Faber. It's available from Milwaukee Pain Clinic, Wm. J. Faber, 6529 W. Fond du Lac Ave., Milwaukee, WI 53218. For more information or a listing of doctors using this method you may contact me. - Mrs. Henry Swantz, Rt. 1, Jamesport, MO 64648.

(Turn to Page 213 before contacting these people.)

JAW INFECTION, HEARING LOSS & CRIPPLING KNEE PROBLEMS

Arthur Heinig
4565 Hwy B.
Land O'Lakes, WI 54540
715-547-3686

I have had knee pain for a couple of years and have a difficult time standing or walking.

I saw another M.D. and he told me to take aspirin and learn to live with the pain. I also have a hearing problem.

After coming to Milwaukee Pain Clinic my hearing has improved — I now have less pain in my leg and more endurance.

I will talk to anyone that calls me. You may publish my story.

Arthur Heinig

FOOT PAIN & INABILITY TO WALK DUE TO DEGENERATIVE JOINT DISEASE

Renee Finkin
82-55 242 Str.
Bellerose, NY 11426

I had surgery on my foot before and in 1990 I had pains in my knee. When I walked I had problems. I could not walk at all. I had to have help with housework. I went to different chiropractor — it was awful. I was in a walker — I could not walk. One step at a time — really slow. Chiropractor gave me hot packs — did help a little — hardly at all.

I read in National Health about Dr. Faber. I wanted something safe and natural.

(Turn to Page 213 before contacting these people.)

In July, 1990 I came to Milwaukee Pain Clinic. In July I could not bend or stand on my own feet. They got me a wheelchair at the airport and I came to the Clinic in a wheelchair.

Dr. Faber saw me and said I was almost bed ridden and that "I had come in time." Dr. Faber gave me some injections and in 4 months the pain went away. It was the first time I could walk across the room. I continued for 3 weeks and I was standing better, walking better and I can spend more time in the shopping mall. "It's wonderful" I can shop for clothes etc. I can clean my own house, shop for food, and fix meals, happier than in a long time.

I would highly recommend Dr. Faber to anyone that contacts me. He literally saved my life.

I would be honored to have you publish my story - It would be wonderful.

Love You, Dr. Faber
Renee Finkin

SEVERE KNEE AND BACK DEGENERATION AND PAIN

Mary Tunkieicz
8410 W. 60th St.
Kenosha, WI 53144
414-654-8398

I have had pain in both knees for a long time, very hard to walk or bend knees. Other clinics told me to have a surgery on both knees. After treatment at Milwaukee Pain Clinic walking became easier, less burning sensation, feel firmer, more stability and can bend knee further.

You may use my story. Others may call at anytime.

Mary Tunkieicz

(Turn to Page 213 before contacting these people.)

20 YEARS OF BACK PAIN AND COULDN'T BREATH THROUGH NOSE

George Wald
5425 Burton Rd.
North Almsted, Ohio 44070
Tel: 216-777-6361

I have had back pain for 24 years. About 22 years ago I went to Chiropractor, and he helped a little. Went to him about 1 1/2 years. About 12 years ago my back kicked up again and I went to Chiropractor again. At this time my hip gave out and I had a hip replacement.

About 3 years ago my back started to hurt and since I belong to National Health Federation. I saw an article in the bulletin, and I heard Dr. Faber lecture in Chicago. I then went back to a Chiropractor. Helped fairly well. My back hurt so bad that in June 1990 I called Dr. Faber.

Neural-fascial therapy has allowed me to breathe through my nose instantly which I couldn't do for at least 20 years.

Since taking treatments with Dr. Faber, my back has gotten progressively better. I have no pain in my back now and I square dance 3 times a week.

I will be glad to talk to anyone and tell them how pleased I am with my treatments at the Milwaukee Pain Clinic.

You may publish my story.

George Wald

(Turn to Page 213 before contacting these people.)

OVER 40 YEARS OF SHOULDER PAIN INSTANT IMPROVEMENT

Bruce Klingkammer
N81 W 13379 Fond du Lac Ave.
Menomonee Falls, WI 53051

I was playing football in high school and the army. Only thing that bothered me was I could not throw. I have had pain for 40 years, but the last 10 years has been bad.

Chiropractor told patient about all he could do for him to help the pain, was to learn to live with it.

After treatment at Milwaukee Pain Clinic, I can now raise my arm higher. I can get my arm up to shave myself. I had trouble putting my shirt on and off and now it is easier. After first treatment, I noticed relief from pain.

Anyone may call me and I will tell them how I have progressed since treatment at Milwaukee Pain Clinic.

You may publish my story.

Bruce Kingkammer

OVER 40 YEARS OF BACK & NECK PROBLEMS

Ben Finkin
82-55 242 St.
Bellerose, NY 11426

When I was a young man, I was involved in an automobile accident. Since then the pain increased slowly in my back. I had whiplash. I went for Chiropractor care for long time. I was bed ridden for 1 whole month, 20 years ago. I was never free from pain, it was continual. I work in construction and movements caused continual pain.

When I heard about Dr. Faber, then I thought of my wife,

(Turn to Page 213 before contacting these people.)

that she needed more care than I did. I thought maybe he could help me, too. Dr. Faber started treatment on me and I had instant relief. I made 1 mistake when I tried to push a refrigerator and some of the pain came back again. I came to Dr. Faber for treatment. I'm so much better now.

I am almost 90% free of pain now and I bless Dr. Faber for the treatments.

I would gladly respond to anyone that contacts me. I call Dr. Faber the "8th wonder of the world." He is really a great doctor.

I would proud for you to publish my story. I would be very flattered.

Ben Finkin

CHRONIC KNEES AND FEET PROBLEMS

Sarah Miller
R. 2 Box 71
Kalona, IA 52247
319-656-2702

Since a couple of years, my knees felt weak. I had a spur on the one knee.

I could not squat down to pick strawberries anymore for many years. Had X-rays and discovered the spur.

I came to the Milwaukee Pain Clinic and I got almost immediate relief from the injections Dr. Faber gave me. My knee really feels great now. I will be glad to talk to anyone about the treatments and relief I got at the Milwaukee Pain Clinic.

You may publish my story.

Mrs. Edward F. Miller

(Turn to Page 213 before contacting these people.)

HEARING LOSS RESTORED

Audrey Christensen
W. 2290 W. 106 Hwy.
Jefferson, WI 53549
Tel: 1-593-2587

About 10 years ago I experienced some hearing loss in my left ear.

I went to several doctors and I was told that there was nothing wrong with my ear. Another doctor suggested a hearing aid, which I got. I was not completely satisfied.

I then came to the Milwaukee Pain Clinic and Dr. Faber injected my ears and head and my hearing was returned. I do not wear my hearing aid at all now.

I would be happy to talk to anyone about how pleased I am with my treatment at Milwaukee Pain Clinic and how my hearing has improved.

You certainly may publish my story.

Audrey Christensen

MULTIPLE KNEE SURGERIES AND WRIST INSTABILITY

Dr. William Revenaugh
38500 Rt. 45
Mellburn, IL 60083
Tel: 708-356-3023

My left knee was operated in the lateral in 1961 - from a ski accident. It started to give me trouble in Spring of 1990 and surgery on it was not successful.

I had surgery on my right knee in 1978 and they put pins in the leg. I then had arthoscopic surgery in 1988. I could

(Turn to Page 213 before contacting these people.)

walk but I could not ski. I had a lot of pain.

I was referred to Dr. Faber by a friend and I came to the Milwaukee Pain Clinic. I saw Dr. Faber and he started treating my knees. The alternative was to have artificial knees put in. Since starting treatment at Milwaukee Pain Clinic, my pain is less, it is now easier to stand after sitting and I can straighten my knees out with less pain. I'm X country skiing again.

I would be glad to talk to anyone who calls me - I'm very satisfied with my treatments.

You may publish my story.

William Revenaugh

SEVERE SPINAL PAIN, GROIN & HIP PAIN

Ed Merck
28 Elm Str.
Norton, MA 02766
508-285-4625

About 6 years ago pain started in my back, some smaller ligament were sprained. I saw many A.M.A. doctors plus massage, rolfing, meditation, and stretching with no relief. I had headaches and stiffness and pain in back and pain on side of left hip and into the calf. I also had Chiropractic treatments. None of this was lasting relief. The doctors did not help at all.

I started treatments at the Milwaukee Pain Clinic and have noticed increased strength, and endurance, less pain and no more spasms. I would be happy to discuss the treatments at Milwaukee Pain Clinic with anyone.

May publish my story.

Ed Merck

(Turn to Page 213 before contacting these people.)

RECOMMENDED RIGHT AND LEFT KNEE REPLACEMENT SURGERY

Floyd Myers
2720 Dougall Str.
Joliet, IL 60432
815-722-0266

My knee problems started 20 years ago. Then about 15 years ago, when I came in from work, and my knees were so swollen. Then in 1981 I could not get up and down which resulted in my changing profession. For the last 5 years I had trouble getting around. Previous doctors told me my knees were wearing out and I would have to have surgery.

Since treatment at Milwaukee Pain Clinic, I have more stamina, do not walk stiff-legged, knees do not "jump out." I can now go up and down steps with ease.

People can call me and I will tell them how happy I am with the treatment.

You may publish my story.

Floyd Myers

This patient was advised to have 2 knee replacements, With reconstruction therapy he cancelled his surgery time for good!

SEVERE CRIPPLING SPINAL PAIN AND HIDDEN JAW & TOOTH PROBLEMS

James Obrzut
405 N. Wabash Ave.
Chicago, IL 60611
Tel: 708-655-9252

I have had constant pain since December of 1987. I was

(Turn to Page 213 before contacting these people.)

lifting a large item and slipped getting out of the car. While trying to hold on to the table, I tore ligaments in my back.

I went to 5 different doctors and they prescribed muscle relaxers, pain pills and anti-inflamatory drugs. These masked some of the pain but I was still in severe pain and spending every minute of my time in bed. I was not able to sit and walked hunched over.

The fifth doctor wanted me to see a psychiatrist, he said it "was all in my head." I then went to see a Chiropractor. Had X-ray, and they showed bulging disc and degenerative disc. I had 65-70 visits to Chiropractor over a 6 months period. He got me physically functioning again, reached a point where Chiropractor sessions were doing me more harm than good.

At that point I came to Milwaukee Pain Clinic and Dr. Faber diagnosed ligament damage all the way up the spine and hips. For 10 years I could not sit even in a car. Dr. Faber was the first to diagnose that my hips needed treatment. I feel this is how my back problem started. I had had a skiing accident and no one bothered to look at the spine.

The treatments Dr. Faber gave me were not progressing as fast as Dr. Faber would like and at this point Dr. Faber sent me to have my mouth X-rayed. They found 5 infected teeth. The infection was so deep under the root canal I had to have separate surgery for that.

I was also fighting a yeast problem and Dr. Faber was the first to diagnose that. Dr. Faber put me on a strict diet. This is now under control by diet and natural supplements. I also had Colonic treatments.

I had minor improvement in pain after the 3rd series of injection. I would say I have improved, and can now sit on a bus and a chair. I had to lift myself by my arm causing

(Turn to Page 213 before contacting these people.)

more strain, now I do not have to do that.

Dr. Faber is now treating my spine. I finished the Sacro treatments after 12 treatments. Still working on lower back and spine. There is a marked improvement.

Anyone may call me and you may publish my story.

James G. Obrzut

26 YEARS OF HERNIATED DISC PROBLEMS ELIMINATED

Ervin Nowak
6015 Briar Clift Court
Greendale, WI 53129
Tel: 414-423-1212

I came to the Milwaukee Pain Clinic because I had a back problem and I heard Dr. Faber on the radio on station WTMJ, and called for an appointment even before he was through talking.

I went to the Milwaukee Pain Clinic and Dr. Faber examined me and sent me for X-rays. He explained the injection therapy to me after he examined my spine. He seemed to know exactly where the problem areas were.

I started the injection therapy and also had some manipulations. After the first treatment, I did have a different feeling in the problem areas. I was really shocked. After that, I had my ups and downs but I continued with the treatments. There was a continuous improvement. I got progressively better. I looked forward to each treatment because of the steady progress and I was rewarded with less pain. At present time my back is feeling very good.

I am very impressed with the Milwaukee Pain Clinic, Dr. Faber and all the friendly people that work there.

I've suffered severe back pain for 26 years. I've had a

(Turn to Page 213 before contacting these people.)

number of admissions to hospital for traction, drugs and had been recommended by 5 surgeons to have ruptured discs removed. I can now do heavy yard work, lift heavy 75 pound bags and not have back pain. I recommend reconstruction/ neural therapy for anyone not finding relief.

I will be most happy to discuss my treatments with anyone that calls me.

You may publish my story.

Ervin Nowak

SEVERE NECK AND HAND PROBLEMS

Lia Corinth
124 Keeney
Evanston, IL 60202
708-328-4202

I went to a lecture that Dr. William Faber presented and the symptoms he described as torn ligaments related to me. His lecture convinced me I was a good candidate for the injection therapy that Dr. Faber described and that it was a superior form of treatment.

Because the ligaments in my neck were wrecked due to a car accident and from the 3 falls off of horses as a teenager, I felt I needed the treatments.

I came to Milwaukee Pain Clinic and started the injection therapy and the pain went away after the first treatment. I had been in severe and constant pain for a long time. After the first treatment I could tell that my neck felt stronger.

I also had lost 30% of the sensation in my hands and did not know it. As the treatments progressed my hands "woke up." As the treatment continued on my neck, I can now look up at the ceiling which I had been unable to do. I always had to hold my head up with my hand before.

(Turn to Page 213 before contacting these people.)

At the Milwaukee Pain Clinic Dr. Faber uses a superior science and it is truly a miracle.

At any time, I will be glad to discuss the treatments I received at Milwaukee Pain Clinic. I have already told many people about the clinic.

You may publish my story.

Lia Corinth

CHRONIC BACK PAIN

James Golick
804 Colfax
Elmhurst, IL 60126
Tel: 708-941-7345

I have had low back pain since age 17. I had, on 6 or 7 occasions, severe back pain which required bed rests and chiropractic adjustments. I got some relief but nothing permanent. I had a herniated disc in November that had me bed ridden for 2 weeks - I am a traveling salesman and had an aggravation of my condition that ended me up in bed for 3 more days.

I made a decision that if I were continue my work as a salesman, I had to get some permanent relief. I heard about the Milwaukee Pain Clinic from a friend, so I decided to call for an appointment at the Milwaukee Pain Clinic. Five days after my first treatment both my chiropractor and I noticed improvement in my back and neck. I can now travel the state and not even a thought about my back.

This is the greatest thing around as Dr. Faber has a fantastic method in the injection therapy. Thank God for Dr. Faber. I will be happy to discuss my treatments with anyone that calls.

(Turn to Page 213 before contacting these people.)

It is so great not to have to worry about my back giving me problems.

You may publish my story.

James Golick

CHRONIC BACK & HIP PAIN

James Hanapel
5445 N. Sheridan Apt. 3312
Chicago, IL 60640
Tel: 312-561-9724

For about 1 1/2 years I had pain in my back and right hip. This was from a fall I took out of a tree when I was about 10 years old.

I heard about the Milwaukee Pain Clinic from a neighbor, they lent me a copy of Dr. Faber's book — Pain, Pain, Go Away. I was very skeptical but I called and made an appointment to see Dr. Faber. I thought I was headed for a wheelchair or a hip replacement.

Dr. Faber started the injection therapy and I had immediate relief - the pain was considerably less. I am very happy with my treatment at Milwaukee Pain Clinic.

I will be more than happy to discuss with anyone my treatments by Dr. Faber.

You may publish my story.

James Hanapel

(Turn to Page 213 before contacting these people.)

CHRONIC SHOULDER PAIN

Leland Wolfe
W 263 S 8575 Oakdale Dr.
Mukwonago, WI 53149
Tel: 662-2094

I have had pain for about 4 months in my left shoulder from throwing some brush away. I went to chiropractor but I only got temporary relief. They could offer nothing permanent.

I heard Dr. Faber from the Milwaukee Pain Clinic on WTMJ and I then bought the book Pain, Pain Go Away, and read it. I decided to call for an appointment to see Dr. Faber and I started the Injection Therapy. I got almost immediate relief from pain in my shoulder. How good it felt.

I definitely found the Milwaukee Pain Clinic to give great results. I would be happy to discuss my treatment with anyone that calls me .

You may publish my story.

Leland E. Wolfe

HEARING PROBLEM

Thomas Laird
4308 N. 88th St.
Milwaukee, WI 53222
414-637-4108

I had been referred to Dr. Spaeth by Dr. Faber from the Milwaukee Pain Clinic. Dr. Spaeth discovered infected cysts in the upper and lower jaw on both sides.

After the first treatment which was the most severely damaged side, I had surgery on my jaw to clean the infection.

(Turn to Page 213 before contacting these people.)

After the jaw surgery, as I was walking home, I felt a click in my right jaw and I had a funny feeling in my head. After 5 minutes or so I realized that I was experiencing normal hearing in the right ear for the first time in perhaps 12 to 15 years. Although I was not deaf, the hearing level had diminished so that I was unable to hear a normal telephone conversation in the right ear. After the surgery I was able to hear the telephone in the right ear. I called all my friends to tell them about it.

I am extremely satisfied with the services rendered by Dr. Spaeth and I am delighted that Dr. Faber referred me to him. After my surgery on the left side of the jaw, the sick feeling I had had for 5 to 6 weeks, went away.

I think Dr. Faber is just great and on to some therapy techniques that are badly needed.

I would be happy to recommend the treatments I have received with anyone that is contemplating the conventional treatment.

You may publish my story.

Thomas G. Laird

HIP DEFORMITY AND PAIN

Dan Chapman
E1200 N
P.O. Box 265
Grant Park, IL 60940
(815) 465-2279

At age 12 I was pole vaulting, missed the mat and fell on my left hip. I never had it looked at by a doctor. It was fine until a year later. I started to play basketball in 8th grade and had pain whenever I played.

I went to several doctors and they did not do X-rays or do anything. When I was in 8th grade I had an X-ray taken and

(Turn to Page 213 before contacting these people.)

they found the cracked bone in my hip. They found the femur bone was not in the socket. I had been going to different doctors and chiropractors and they were not doing any good. They told me to wait and they could put in a plastic hip. I tried reflexology and that did not help.

From 7th grade to 10th grade I had pain in my hip. I enjoy sports but I could not run as fast as everyone else did. At one point the pain did let up a little but still hurt at night and I was extremely weak.

My mother read Dr. Faber's book Pain, Pain Go Away and I read it. I was very apprehensive about coming to the Pain Clinic but my mother called for an appointment for me. I talked to Dr. Faber and I started the injection therapy. I had a lot of relief after the 2nd treatment and each treatment is so much better. I now have no pain.

The Milwaukee Pain Clinic is a dream come true. I will discuss my treatments with anyone that calls.

You may publish my story.

Dan Chapman

CHRONIC HIP AND LOW BACK PAIN

Ruth Ann Hansen
418 Winnebago
Park Forest, IL 60466
708-748-5653

I have had pain in my hip and low back area for about 5 years, gradually getting worse.

I tried Chiropractor treatment for about 1 year but the treatments did not bring much relief.

I belong to the Natural Health Federation and I heard Dr. Faber talk. I was looking for something for relief of pain, and I decided to call the Milwaukee Pain Clinic.

(Turn to Page 213 before contacting these people.)

I had almost immediate relief of pain and gradually I could space my visits to the Milwaukee Pain Clinic.
I did not want to go through any surgery and I wanted some treatment that was more natural. This was a totally different feeling for me and I enjoyed coming to the Milwaukee Pain Clinic.

The treatments at the Clinic are of such a positive attitude. My relationship with Dr. Faber is so great. I know the treatment I am getting will produce good results. Other doctors always gave me the feeling that I did not know anything and the feeling that Dr. Faber expressed to me was so positive.

I will be glad to discuss my treatments with anyone that calls me.

You may publish my story.

Ruth Hansen

CHRONIC HEAD, NECK & BACK PAIN

Barbara Zuzanek
112 Hickary Rd.
Gary, IL 60013
708-516-1225

I had an automobile accident about 10 years ago and I was thrown out of my jeep, hanging by my seat belt. I was taken to the hospital and the doctor told me there was nothing wrong with me except a cracked rib. I was black and blue from my face down.

Through the years I lived on aspirin, but I noticed every night my back was hurting. It got to the point where the pain in my back would not go away. Five years went by with all this pain.

(Turn to Page 213 before contacting these people.)

Then, my dentist recommended that I see Chiropractor and I went to see the Chiropractor for about 4 years. For awhile these treatments helped but I was never free of pain. Then, the pain steadily got worse and I was getting no relief at all.

My husband recommended that I go to see a Physical Therapist to see what he could do for me. By this time I was taking 100 aspirin tablets a week with no relief. I went to Physical Therapy for 1 year but it was not helping and my tail bone, hip and neck would not stay in place. They kept rotating out of place. The aspirin bottle and I were still good friends. I was afraid to do anything for fear it would make something move out of place. I could hardly walk up the stairs, get out of bed or ride in the car. The every day household chores hurt so much to do.

Then, I started to read Dr. William Faber of the Milwaukee Pain Clinic book, and I could not put it down until I finished it at midnight. I could hardly wait until morning to call for an appointment. I figured I had nothing to lose and everything to gain - so why not?

And, have I gained - after my first treatment I had immediate relief from my constant headaches and within 24 hours my headaches had not returned. The dizziness I had for years also disappeared. The pain in my back is disappearing and keeps getting better all the time.

I feel happy again and I can now do my household chores and cook meals.

In fact, I look forward to my treatments every week because I continue to improve. It is so hard to believe that after living with the terrible pain I had I am actually 80 % improved and I'm shooting for 100 %.

I still get scared at times, if I make a sudden move, make a bed or vacuuming that I'll start to hurt again. But, I'm finding that as each day goes by I'm not hurting. It is so wonderful to get up and not go for the aspirin bottle.

I don't know how to thank Dr. Faber for all the good he

(Turn to Page 213 before contacting these people.)

has done for me, except to tell other people like me "Quit fooling around," get some relief at the Milwaukee Pain Clinic. You do not need to keep hurting day after day. Do something about it. If it can work for me, it can work for you.

I'll be happy to hear from you and tell you personally how Dr. Faber helped me.

You may publish my story.

Barbara Zuzanek

CHRONIC NOSE, NECK AND SHOULDER PAIN

Donald Schnack
2021 Rhode Island Ave., N.
Minneapolis, Minn. 55427
612-544-3474

As the result of a car accident in 1989, I started to have pain in my neck, shoulders, and right upper arm, numbness in forefinger and thumb on my right hand, sharp pain in the shoulder blade across the right arm and down into the elbow. I could not put my right arm behind my back. Not being able to bring my right arm behind me, past vertical body line, I could not hook up my seat belt. I could not shift by 5 speed Mazda into reverse.

I started taking chiropractic treatments three times weekly. I went to see a neurosurgeon, orthopaedic surgeon, had massage therapy, CT scan, MRI, electronic nerve evaluation and these treatments were all in vain.

The suggestion of neck surgery and the thought of my having my throat cut from ear to ear did not agree with me. I was told "I would just have to live with the pain." This was a poor alternative for me to accept. Besides, the possible degree of success of the surgery did not bring about a state of euphoria. I just knew there had to be an alternative so I

(Turn to Page 213 before contacting these people.)

steadfastly denied the surgery.

Not being able to sleep, only 40 minutes to an hour at a time since the accident, had taken it's toll. I could adjust to some of the pain with the help of a "TENS Unit" and a portable vertical traction device, along with frequent chiropractic adjustments. The loss of sleep really affected my life.

Fortunately, some friends of mine from Minneapolis told me of their success at the Milwaukee Pain Clinic, so without a moment's hesitation I made an appointment to see Dr. William Faber.

The 360 mile drive passed quickly because of the excitement and anticipation of NO PAIN.

Because metabolic efficiency had been my life style for many years, the results of my first injection therapy were very favorable and exceeded my expectations. From my friend from Minnesota to Dr. Faber gave me instantaneous relief. Was there total relief of pain and did I have complete range of motion? No, but I did not expect this. However, I immediately knew that my prayers had been answered. I can now bring my arm behind me, moments after the first treatment. Not all the way, but it is a start.

Today, 16 months after my accident, I am confident I am on the road to recovery. I have nearly full range of motion, I can sleep 3-4 hours without waking to the severe pain in my shoulders, arms, and the low grade headache at the base of my skull. The numbness in my thumb and forefinger while driving does not occur.

I have just completed my 5th treatment and for a 65 year old, it is pretty exciting to be free of pain and mobile. I now know that total pain elimination and full mobility is just over the horizon.

I will gladly discuss my treatments with anyone that calls me. You may publish my story.

Donald Schnack

(Turn to Page 213 before contacting these people.)

CHRONIC DIZZINESS AND NECK PAIN

Suzanne Schweiger
1614 N. Yale
Arlington Heights, Ill 60004
312-394-8792

I fell off a hay ride in October of 1976, and about 2 weeks after that I started getting a off balance feeling. I went to Chiropractor and they could not help me. I also saw Osteopathic doctors with little results.

I heard that Dr. Faber from Milwaukee Pain Clinic was going to give a presentation at Niles, Illinois Library and I decided to attend. I called and made an appointment. Changing doctors had always been scary to me but I found Dr. Faber to be a recommendable doctor. I started the Injection Therapy and I was surprised that I noticed immediate relief from the pain. I had had severe jaw pain and the injections "took care of that." I feel the Milwaukee Pain Clinic and Dr. Faber saved my life.

I would gladly discuss my treatment at the Clinic.

You may publish my story.

Suzanne Schweiger

FAILED SPINAL SURGERY

Philip Strohm
316 Woodland Beach Rd.
Lake Mills, WI 53551
414-648-5280

I have had back trouble almost all of my life, even back in grade school I had problems.

I went to Chiropractors through the years and the relief

(Turn to Page 213 before contacting these people.)

I got would not last. Around 1955 the pain got so bad, that I had to go in for surgery and I had a Laminectomy. I got some relief but I had to wear a brace. The doctors told me everybody has a little pain in their life and you will have to learn to relax and live with the pain.

About 8 years ago I went to an Orthopedic doctor, he X-rayed and told me "I wouldn't touch you surgery wise." "Learn to live with the pain." About June of '89, it got so bad I could not stand the pain. I went to a different Orthopedic doctor and he said my lamina were rubbing on one another. Dr. removed those and I felt better, but still had pain.

I was listening to W.T.M.J. and I heard Dr. Faber talk about back problems and he said Reconstruction therapy could strengthen the ligaments and muscles. I immediately bought Dr. Faber's book — Pain, Pain Go Away and it made so much sense to me. I then called for an appointment and came to see Dr. Faber.

I was so surprised I had almost immediate relief from my pain. I was so impressed with the immediate results I obtained. It defied my understanding of the injection therapy. I am so happy with my progress. My back feels so much firmer and I have much more strength - I feel it is here to stay.

I would be happy to talk to anyone that calls me. All my friends have been told about my treatments.

You may publish my story.

Philip A. Strohm

FAILED NECK & BACK SURGERY

John Parks Trowbridge, M.D.

At age 14 I was running track and developed low back pain. I started seeing a chiropractor 1 to 2 times a week for

(Turn to Page 213 before contacting these people.)

5 years. It helped and kept me going but didn't alter the course of constant aching, pulling, nagging back pain. When a junior in college after moving furniture I went as an emergency to a medical center and was told I had degenerative disc and inflammation of L4-5 and L5-S1 discs. They gave rest, exercise, Tylenol #3, Darvon Compound-65, Indocin and Butazoylidin alka. These medications fogged my brain and gave me G.I. upset. They didn't change the course of the now daily back pain.

At age 23 on a trip to San Diego, I dove into the hotel swimming pool's cold water. It triggered muscle spasms and I then got severe sciatica down my left leg. I didn't know if I could swim to the side. I struggled out of the pool and literally crawled in agony to the hotel room. I took the most painful ride of my life lying in the back of a volkswagon Beetle 500 miles to my home in Stanford, California. My orthopedist gave Demoral injections, Tylenol #3, muscle-relaxant and anti-inflammatory drugs. I was in bed two weeks. I saw a chiropractor as I could afford it. Six months later I picked up a pencil and all my sciatic pain returned with a vengeance. This time medications were repeated as before and another 3 weeks flat on my back. The next several years involved more chiropractic, exercise and drugs. Sometimes I'd just sneeze and have to go down for a day or two.

In April 1979 while moving into a new house I sprained my neck. It just worsened the next week. Then I lost grasp of my left hand. I was admitted for a week of therapy. I got better, went back to work and then it happened again. Finally on 6-19-79 had a cervical laminectomy at C-5-6 on the left. I had a long and painful post-up recovery wearing a hard cervical collar for 2 months. I just started in my first practice as a solo general practitioner in November 1978. I was broke. Everything was very hard. Our budget allowed only for food and gas. My surgery caused me to start my

(Turn to Page 213 before contacting these people.)

practice all over again. My recovery left me with a residual numbness, tingling and occasional sharp pain in the forearm and fingers for several years. One thing I didn't mention was that the cervical myelogram activated my sciatic pain once again. I clearly recall begging my surgeon to operate on my low back at the same time. My life continued to deteriorate. If I did any activity like vacuuming, carring groceries I dearly paid for it. I'd grit my teeth to get through each day. I only did what I had to do to get through each day. My wife would like to visit her family 3 to 6 hours away, the ride would cause activation of my sciatica for 2 days each way. Even airplane flight would aggravate my back and leg pain.

In November, Thanksgiving 1988 I went bowling at my sister-in-laws. I slipped with the ball and fell. I awakened with increasing low back pain. The following week I just had worse left sciatica. I called my neurosurgeon friend who got me a magnetic resonance scan on 12/7/88. The report was complete herniated disc L4-5 on the left. I had x-rays, cat scan and myelogram on hospital admission. My neurosurgeon said "I love patient's like you, I like my residents to see real pathology." Emergency surgery was performed that afternoon. I awoke the next morning without pain. I was discharged 2 days later and in another 2 days was back to work. This surgery was a snap compared to my first spinal surgery. All went well until putting on my cowboy boots for "Go Texan Day!" in late February 1989. I got a sudden stabbing low back pain. I went to my pharmacy for pain and muscle relaxers. I put my back brace on. For over the next year I had the feeling my back was unstable. It would just slip and bite. On April 10, 1990 packing for a trip it went crazy on me again.

The next months it caused increasing pain in my back and leg. I had to be very careful and still had pain just turning over in bed. I interviewed Dr. Bill Faber for my syndicated 150 station radio show "Finally Feeling Better."

(Turn to Page 213 before contacting these people.)

Reading Pain, Pain Go Away in preparation for the show revealed that finally someone understood precisely what my problem was and had the ideal solution. I committed myself to getting reconstruction and neural fascial therapy. I made my phone arrangements and Dr. Faber treated me carefully from head to foot after reviewing my entire life history. Immediately I could tell the deep aching pain was relieved in my back and leg. I took my plane trips without near as much discomfort as before. I noticed over days my neck and back strengthening. I had for the first time more confidence in getting out of cars and chairs. I was actually excited and couldn't wait to fly back for more treatments.

The following treatments provided more relief to the previous. I could now lift my 23 lb 2 years old daughter with much more comfort. I don't need as many chiropractic treatments. I have not needed any medications since my first treatments. After my second treatment I realized I must take Dr. Faber's preceptorship course so that these wonderful therapies can me more available to chronic pain which I knew so well.

At the time of this writing I've had only 3 sessions of neural/fascial - reconstruction therapy I know that I'll never relapse which was my mode of living for 25 years. The strength, endurance and confidence in my spine is clearly evident to me. I drive 6-8 hours to visit and don't have the deep aching I knew for so long.

I would recommend the non-surgical neural-fascial reconstruction method over surgery or any other technique for chronic spinal disc pain. My back and neck are truly better in every single way as a direct result of these wonderful but powerful tiny injection treatments. I anticipate over time a total permanent recovery. I am doing everything in my power to clear my schedule and complete the preceptorship training in the summer of 1991. If you wish a verification of

(Turn to Page 213 before contacting these people.)

this statement please send self-addressed legal sized stamped envelope to me. Or if you wish call office at 1-800-2HELP-YOU.

John Parks Trowbridge M.D.
9816 Memorial Blvd. Ste. 205
Humble,Texas 77338
Author - The Yeast Syndrome,
President-Elect, The American Academy
for the Advancement of Medicine

WRIST INSTABILITY RESOLVED

Dr. Gary Anderson D.C.
3299 Miller
Bethany, MO 64424
816-425-3738

I developed pain, swelling and constant aching in my wrists from doing Chiropractic adjustments. I had adjustments to my neck and wrists, took nutritional supplements. These all failed to produce adequate results. This problem has plagued me for over five years. I was beginning to think, "What am I going to when I couldn't give hand adjustments anymore." Dr. Bill's reconstruction therapy gave me strength and endurance to my wrists again. My years of pain and swelling are gone for good. In fact, I don't even think of my wrist anymore.

If anyone wishes to contact me for verification of this story, I'll be happy to tell them of reconstruction/neural therapy's tremendous healing benefits.

(Turn to Page 213 before contacting these people.)

SEVERE NECK, BACK AND TMJ

Charles Stepanek
420 S. Victoria Circle
New Berlin, WI 53151
414-797-0978

I had severe neck and back pain and in the sciatica. I could not turn my head or hold my head up. I had pain in my left leg. The sciatic pain was like a jolt of lightning going thru my body. I had this pain for about 8 months. I had sought treatment else where without any success.

I came to the Milwaukee Pain Clinic after the family doctor recommended I go the Mayo Clinic but I would not accept the idea of surgery. I listened to Dr. Faber lecture and decided this was my only hope. Dr. Faber started the injections in my neck because I could not sit up in a chair. From there, Dr. Faber gave me therapy up and down my spine. I have gotten progressively better and I feel like a human being again. The pain has subsided in all area.

If it wasn't for the Milwaukee Pain Clinic, I would have had to go to Mexico for treatment. Dr. Faber is so interested in his patients health. Unfortunately there are not enough Doctors like him around.

I will gladly talk to anyone that has the same pain problems I have.

You may publish my story.

Charles Stepanek

(Turn to Page 213 before contacting these people.)

FAILED SPINAL SURGERY

Warren Tabor
8513 Meadow Lake Pl.
New Hope, Minn 54428
612-533-9327

Eight years ago I had lower back surgery and that was for Stenosis — a pressure on nerves between vertebrae. — This fall, I injured my back — compressed it more, by heavy lifting. I thought I would have to live with the pain.

Mrs. Boyd's son had contact with Dr. Faber and he reported Milwaukee Pain Clinic to be a source of help to her knee. Due to the fact my back was hurting and my wife's neck was in pain, we decided to come to see Dr. Faber.

We came to get treatment from Dr. Faber. After just 10 treatments of injection therapy most of the pain is gone. I did some more heavy lifting and I re-injured my back, so I came back for more treatments, because I really believe in these treatments.

We were given the confidence in the ability of the clinic to correct the pain we were enduring. The Pain Clinic is great.

I certainly will recommend and talk to anyone that would call me. I have recommended the Milwaukee Pain Clinic to my friends.

The Pain Clinic has so many friendly people.

You may publish my story.

Warren R. Tabor

(Turn to Page 213 before contacting these people.)

SPONDYLOLISTHESIS

Craig A. Ewald
Vice President
Ewald Automotive Group
2201 North Mayfair Rd.
Milwaukee, WI 53226
414-258-5000

To whom it may concern....

Did I have a problem with 24 hour around the clock pain. Over two years of it....

My problem was a lumbar spondylolisthesis. This is a break in the vertebra causing my spine to slip forward off its base. This affected me causing deep aching pain in my low back which worsened with activities. I sought the help of a large well known clinic. They wanted to fuse my back with surgery. I went to Dr. Faber for this problem. He told me reconstruction therapy was better than surgery for my condition. I was not fond of injections but I had seen poor results surgery had given many of my friends. I decided to do reconstruction.

One thing is for certain reconstruction therapy fully restored my back. I can Golf, Waterski, Swim, Hunt, do land scaping (my hobby) and other activities that used to cause me severe pain.

My therapy was completed over 7 years ago. I have had no recurrences. I consider my back reconstructed and cured.

I recommend that people get reconstruction therapy from Dr. Faber after they read his book. I'll be happy to verify this letter to any who wish to call me. If you write please include a self addressed stamped envelope.

Sincerely,
Craig A. Ewald

(Turn to Page 213 before contacting these people.)

FAILED SPINAL DISC SURGERY

Ezell Wilson
539 N. 33rd.
Milwaukee, WI 53208
933-1724

I had a back problem that happened at my work. I couldn't do anything. I had difficulty standing sitting or walking. I had the pain for about 3 years before I discovered the Milwaukee Pain Clinic.

I came to see Dr. Faber and it was decided that I needed Injection therapy. I started taking the injection and in a very short time I noticed marked relief. I continued the treatments and now my back is as solid as a rock.

I am so pleased with my treatment at Milwaukee Pain Clinic because I had been to see 4 other doctors and they told me I had to learn to live with the pain.

I heard the Milwaukee Pain Clinic is a great place to come to get constant release of pain.

If anyone wishes to call me, I will tell them about the great results I obtained at Milwaukee Pain Clinic.

I have had my treatment over 8 years ago. I have had no back problems since.

You may publish my story.

Ezell Wilson

(Turn to Page 213 before contacting these people.)

SEVERE HEAD, NECK AND BACK PAIN

Elaine Steufen
12903 Mississippi Rd.
Elk River, Minn. 55330
612-441-1403

I had an accident 10 years ago and my eyes were blurry, couldn't bend, had a pulling if I tried to lean forward and a jab in the middle of my back.

Two years ago I went to a Chiropractor and he worked on my neck and unjammed the cervical in my neck. My lower back was also jammed and he loosened that too. I had a lot of head pain and pressure and a pain in my arm. I went to the Chiropractor and he adjusted my cervical but it would not stay in place. I was in constant agony. My friend from Elk River was already a patient at the Milwaukee Pain Clinic and she recommended I come to see Dr. Faber.

I made an appointment and Dr. Faber thought I would be a good candidate for the Proliferative Therapy. Dr. Faber started doing the injections on my neck and I found out my back also needed the injections in different areas.

After I started the therapy on my neck, it felt stronger. My back now is being treated and already I have noticed some increase in strength. The Cervicals are holding in place now the pain is a lot less now because I had pain in my neck, throat, head and even my teeth. The pain in my tongue and throat is gone, my head and neck feel very good.

I am so glad I came to the Milwaukee Pain Clinic because it was my last resort.

I would like to help somebody else to feel pain free and will gladly talk to anyone.

You may publish my story.

Elaine Stuefen

(Turn to Page 213 before contacting these people.)

DEFORMED FOOT AND SCOLIOSIS

Diane Remy
Diane Remy School of Dance & Baton
2305 N. 8th
Sheboygan, WI 53083
414-452-8697

I first noticed pain in my feet and ankle about 10 years ago along with a lot of weakness. Since I own my own Dance Studio, I had to depend on my ankle and at this point, I could not do this. I also have a congenital foot deformity.

I contacted other doctors and they all suggested surgery with no guarantee, or learn to live with the condition and I was so afraid I would have to give up my Dancing profession.

In addition, through the years. I have had back problems caused by Scoliosis of the spine.

My mother had attended a workshop of Wisconsin Natural Health Association and she brought me some literature on the Milwaukee Pain Clinic. After I read all this literature, I called the Milwaukee Pain Clinic and made an appointment to see Dr. Faber.

After a consultation with Dr. Faber, it was decided I had to be built up nutritionally and he suggested I have some IV's to do this. After the first month of IV's, Dr. Faber decided to start the Proliferative Therapy. We started the injections on my ankle and gradually my ankle got stronger and firmer. I now had a better range of motion and more flexibility plus feeling stronger. The muscle spasms have disappeared and I can now rely on my back not to give out when I am teaching dancing.

Since dancing is my life profession I almost had to give it

(Turn to Page 213 before contacting these people.)

up. Thank goodness, I found the Milwaukee Pain Clinic.

I am so happy to have found a place like the Milwaukee Pain Clinic or I don't know what I would have done.

The pain in my foot has lessened. I am much sharper mentally and I do not get so tired any more.

I will be happy to share my experience at Milwaukee Pain Clinic. I will discuss this with anyone that calls me.

You may publish my story.

Diane Remy

CHRONIC KNEE PAIN

Paul F. Reifsteck
552 Gulch Ave.
Wisconsin Dells, WI 53965
608-254-8284

About 6 years ago I ran out of my house to shut of a motor and I turned my knee, then about 6-8 months ago I had pain in my knee come on gradually.

I saw several doctors and was not satisfied with their diagnosis. Since I belong to the National Health Federation. I discovered an ad in their newspaper telling about the Milwaukee Pain Clinic.

I called Dr. Faber and made an appointment to see him and I started the injection therapy. I have had continued improvement in my knee since starting the treatments.

The Milwaukee Pain Clinic is great and the first place to go for ligament damage since I firmly believe in natural healing.

I have talked to many people about how wonderful I feel

(Turn to Page 213 before contacting these people.)

about my recovery and I certainly will talk to anyone that contacts me.

You may publish my story.

Paul F. Reifsteck

TORN KNEE CARTILAGE

Steven Siehr
47 S. Main
Fond du Lac, WI 54935
923-1779

I tore the cartilage in my knee last February but I felt the knee start to loosen up for one and half years before I tore the cartilage. I had seen orthopedic doctors and they advised surgery. I had had an MRI and they found the torn cartilage.

I started collecting information, and a friend of mine, another artist, has had treatments at Milwaukee Pain Clinic. Since this was a different approach, I investigated the treatment, then read the book Pain Pain Go Away and decided to call for an appointment.

Even after my first consultation with Dr. Faber I felt that the injection therapy tightened the ligaments in my knee.I was very surprised that I had instant relief after the first treatment.

Now, before the treatment I had a permanent limp and a really stiff knee. After the first treatment the swelling subsided and right off the bat, I walked without a limp.

The treatment produced instant relief from symptoms of

(Turn to Page 213 before contacting these people.)

injury and allowed the body to heal itself.

I will gladly discuss my treatment with anyone that calls.

You may publish my story.

Steven O. Siehr

SIEHR, Steven O.	MRI-OP	J.A. Welsch MD
47 S. Main St. FDl		39 years
6-26-90	176339	14-82-70

CLINICAL: Trauma 5-28-90. Medial pain. No prior surgery.

LEFT KNEE MRI: Sequences obtained include short TR sagittal, gradient echo sagittal, followed by short TR coronal.

FINDINGS: There is a bucket handle tear, which is quite extensive, involving the posterior horn, body, and posterior aspect of the anterior horn of the medial meniscus.

There is medial displacement of a fragment of the apical region of the body of the meniscus to a point near the intercondylar notch (images 4.07-4.08).

The lateral miniscus is intact. The cruciate ligaments show no definite evidence of disruption.

There is a small effusion.

Osseous structures reveal no evidence of significant bone edema or occult fracture. There are a couple of tiny benign islands of sclerosis, which should be of no clinical significance.

The medial and lateral collateral ligaments show no definite evidence of disruption.

IMPRESSION: Extensive bucket handle tear medial meniscus left knee.

TJA/sms 6-27-90

(Turn to Page 213 before contacting these people.)

CARPAL TUNNEL SYNDROME

Thomas Laird
4308 N. 88th St.
Milwaukee, WI 53222
461-6539

I was having severe pain in my wrists from repeated motions. The orthopedist said you need carpal tunnel surgery.

I got Dr Faber's injections instead. Am I glad. I got more than I dreamed of at the Milwaukee Pain Clinic.

Thomas Laird

National Health Federation
212 W. Foothill Blvd.
Monrovia, CA 91017

To Whom It May Concern:

I recently visited Dr. William Faber at the MILWAUKEE PAIN CLINIC, located in Milwaukee, Wisconsin. My mother, who is 80 years old, was complaining of stiffness and pain in her legs and knees.

Dr. Faber injected her mouth with a solution and, immediately after the injection, she was able to lift her legs and bend her knees without the stiffness and pain. We were amazed with the instant results. Dr. Faber achieved through working with the mouth. She is also able to walk faster and chew better.

Dr. Faber said he is working with the mouth to help other

(Turn to Page 213 before contacting these people.)

areas of the body. I feel this would be a great topic to share at the National Health Federation Conferences as it would be of interest to everyone in the health field.

Sincerely,
Evelyn Slowinski
4901 S. Lamon
Chicago, IL 60638
312-582-3400

E.W. McDonagh, D.O., A.C.G.P
McDonagh Medical Center, Inc.
2800-A Kendallwood Parkway
Kansas City, MO 64119

Joyce Wunder, housewife, age 58

Diagnoses:

1. Diabetes, type II
2. Generalized atherosclerosis
3. Severe degenerative arthritis, right knee for 20 years.

This lady could not stand more than 3 to 5 minutes due to severe right knee pain. She required a four-legged aluminum walker device to get about her house. Pain became constant four months prior to her first treatment here, and her ability to walk drastically reduced. She could not attend church, shop for groceries, etc. Told by two specialists that her only way out of this problem was knee replacement surgery, she came to this clinic for EDTA chelation therapy for her diabetic vascular problems, in preparation for this surgery.

After beginning EDTA therapy she elected to add recon-

(Turn to Page 213 before contacting these people.)

structive joint injection therapy to her treatment regime. She was given multiple small injections of morrhuate sodium proliferating solution into the tendons and ligaments of the knee joint.

After four treatments she discontinued use of the walker device and can walk, stand and shop all day long without pain or limitation. She was given no manipulation, physiotherapy, prescription drugs, physical restriction advice, or any other treatments.

Mr. Houston Haugo, age 48

Diagnoses:
1. Diabetes, type II
2. Peripheral vascular disease of both legs and feet
3. Frozen left foot and ankle

This gentleman, a banker, had broken his right ankle and foot in a skiing accident 6 years before. The bony fragments were surgically pinned and he has had no functional problems with this foot.

The left foot however, had no flexion, extension or lateral rotation, it was frozen. A 3 cm by 6 cm fusiform arthritic calcification was present along the superior medial aspect of this foot. The foot and ankle was cold to touch, and without sensation of pain and proprioception. He complained of left lower leg pain above the ankle.

He began EDTA chelation therapy for his diabetic vascular problems but continued to complain about his left foot and ankle. He exhibited a pronounced limp when walking.

He requested reconstructive injection therapy to his left foot and ankle, and this treatment was added to his program.

(Turn to Page 213 before contacting these people.)

Multiple injections of minute amounts of proliferating solution were given into the ligaments and tendons of the left foot and ankle.

After the second treatment warmth and sensation returned and functional movement was 70 to 75% normal. After the fourth treatment he had normal function, no pain and could walk normally.

He was given no physiotherapy, manipulation, prescription drugs, advice as to physical restriction, or any other treatments.

Mr. Dean Swansen, age 70

Diagnoses:
1. Atherosclerosis
2. Lumber disc compression syndrome
3. Arthritic deterioration and instability of spine

This patient give a history of multiple falls and injuries to his back and hips during his career as a farmer, resulting in spurring, arthritic deterioration, disc compression, and destabilization of the vertebral column. For the past three months prior to his first visit to this clinic, he could not sleep uninterrupted more than one hour due to recurring pain. If he attempted to lay on his left side additional excruciating pain would radiate into his left side additional excruciating pain would radiate into his left side and down the left leg.

He was treated with EDTA chelation therapy for his vascular occlusive disease. In addition he elected to add reconstructive joint injection therapy to his treatment program.

After one treatment of multiple small amounts of the

(Turn to Page 213 before contacting these people.)

proliferating solution into the tendons and ligaments of the dorsal and lumbar spine and sacroiliac joints, he was pain free. He stated the next morning, "Doc, I slept the whole night through."

He was given no prescription drugs, manipulation, physiotherapy, physical restriction advise, or any other treatment.

SEVERE NECK & KNEE PAIN

Della Dobbratz
710 Park St.
Beaver Dam, WI 53716
414-887-2916

I have had pain in my neck for about two years. I sought medical help and the doctors thought I had a muscle pull in my neck plus some arthritis. I had had mastoid surgery and developed a pain in and behind my ear. I saw a physical therapist for three weeks but he said could not help me and that I should learn to sit up straight.

I heard Dr. Faber talk over the radio and I called for an appointment because the pain was getting worse.

At first, Dr. Faber prescribed supplements and referred me to a special dentist, because Dr. Faber thought I had an infection in my jaw bone. I then had the work done on my jaw bone. I started the Injection Therapy in the back of my ear, my head, neck, back and both sides of my spine.

My neck immediately felt stronger but I still had a lot of pain. Since continuing the treatment my head, back and

(Turn to Page 213 before contacting these people.)

neck keep improving with each treatment. My ear lobe was numb from the mastoid surgery and the feeling has started to come back in the ear lobe too, as result of the injections.

My husband is also receiving treatments at the Pain Clinic on his knee and is showing improvement.

I think the Milwaukee Pain Clinic is more thorough than anywhere else.

I tell people about my treatments and have already recommended another patient to the clinic.

You may publish my story.

Della Dobbratz

SHOULDER DISABILITY

Lyle Cherney
Rural Route 1
New London, WI
414-982-5031

I had pain in my shoulder about three years ago and I had to give up bow hunting, which I liked alot.

I had seen several other doctors and they gave me oral drugs. Then cortisone shots and if that didn't work I'd have to have surgery. I did not want that.

I saw an ad about Dr. Faber in the Wisconsin Natural Food Association, and I decided to call for an appointment.

I made an appointment and came to see Dr. Faber at the Milwaukee Pain Clinic. Dr. Faber started to inject the scar area on my stomach, elbow, wrist, arm, toes, and my head.

(Turn to Page 213 before contacting these people.)

I have been hit in the head several times. — Dr. Faber started to inject my shoulder and real soon I felt more mobility and less pain. I can now raise my arm up over my head and I could not do that before.

Dr. Faber called attention to my infected teeth and I had the teeth removed and my jaw bone scraped. My neck pain disappeared after work was done. The general soreness in my neck has gone away.

I appreciate the fact that Dr. Faber looked at the whole body for causes and treated accordingly, rather than just treating the symptoms, as the medical profession does.

I would discuss the treatments that I received at the Pain Clinic with anyone.

You may publish my story.

Lyle Cherney

SEVERE NECK TEARS

Richard Green
2200 Lewis
Zion, IL 60099
708-746-3402

I have had headaches and pain in my entire cervical area for two and a half years. This was from a weight lifting injury.

I saw a neurologist and that doctor performed several nerve tests and said I had a blockage in the neck. This doctor wanted to do a myelogram. I did not want that because I

(Turn to Page 213 before contacting these people.)

knew the next step would be surgery, I then started to see a chiropractor and he had me convinced that I would be cured in a month. The treatments only helped for a short time. There was a nerve blockage, so the headaches became non-stop. I then saw a different chiropractor and he put me in traction, used acupuncture, a cervical collar, electrical muscle stimulation and he convinced me I'd be better in a couple of months. I was not happy with the results, so I sought out a different chiropractor. He offered a different adjustment technique. —This was a Sports Medicine Chiropractor and he convinced me I'd be better in a month. I then took some physical therapy and they recommended I see an Atlas Chiropractor. —This doctor performed a non-force adjustment technique, this technique did have better results, but there was no lasting results.

I sought out another chiropractor and he convinced me I'd be better in a short period of time, his treatment did not help either.

My mother saw Dr. Faber, of the Milwaukee Pain Clinic, on TV and she ordered the book. I read the book and then called for an appointment. Nothing had worked so far and I desperately needed help.

I started the Injection Therapy and stopped seeing the non-force technique chiropractor. After a couple of treatments I could see some good results, with my neck getting firmer. — My cervical area is getting firmer, my headaches are almost gone and my constant fatigue is getting better all the time.

The Milwaukee Pain Clinic is the best place to go after having other forms of therapy that really do not work.

I will gladly tell anyone about my success at Milwaukee Pain Clinic and you may publish my story.

Rich Green

(Turn to Page 213 before contacting these people.)

SEVERE FOOT AND HEEL PAIN

Olive Keller
2911 S. 71st St
Milwaukee, WI 53219
1-541-1367

One day when I went to step on my left foot, I noticed pain in my heel. After about 2 months I went to a foot doctor. He gave me a lot of cortisone shots and taped up my arch. This did not help at all. I went back to the foot doctor and he told me there was nothing he could do about it. At this point I could not walk.

I decided to call Dr. Faber and make an appointment. I had a series of injections right into the heel and the instep plus the ankle. After the 3rd series of injections I began to get relief. I am still continuing the treatments.

I think the Milwaukee Pain Clinic as the only place a person can get true healing. I don't know what I would do without the Pain Clinic.

I will gladly talk to anyone that contacts me. I have already talked to several people about Dr. Faber. If he moves out of town, I will panic.

You may publish my story.

Olive Keller

NECK, ANKLE AND EYE PROBLEMS

Glenn Rysgaard
3254 S. 69th St
Milwaukee, WI 53219
414-543-0950

I twisted my ankle while riding on a horse, and some-

(Turn to Page 213 before contacting these people.)

thing popped in my ankle. The next morning I had alot of pain. I had x-rays taken and the doctor found a sprain in the Achilles tendon.

Through the National Food Association, I heard Dr. Faber talk on the Reconstruction Therapy. I then ordered Dr. Faber's book Pain, Pain Go Away and read it.

I decided to call for any appointment and I started the injection therapy. The pain in my ankle has gotten progressively better and much firmer.

My neck had pain also so Dr. Faber started injecting the neck and I could focus better with both eyes. The numbness in my face went away after several treatments.

The results were spectacular, and I am very happy with my treatment.

I will discuss my treatments with anyone that calls me.

You may publish my story.

Glenn O. Rysgaard

SEVERE BACK AND HIP PAIN

Paul Hauch
225 N. 7th Ave
West Bend, WI 53095
Tel. 414-334-9091

I had pain in my back and hips for close to 30 years. The pain gradually kept getting worse.

I sought help through several chiropractors, getting only temporary relief. The pain always returned. I could hardly walk steps, could do no lifting, and could not do any heavy work.

I saw an ad on TV about the Milwaukee Pain Clinic, and I called for an appointment. I started the injection therapy at the Clinic, and then I also took the Chelation treatment.

(Turn to Page 213 before contacting these people.)

After about 3rd Chelation treatment the pain started to go away. I could now walk steps. I now could do anything I wanted. I now exercise on a treadmill, rowing machine and jog.

I think the Milwaukee Pain Clinic is awesome. I'm so pleased with my treatments and they are permanent.

Anyone may call me and I'll tell them how pleased I am with being pain free.

You may publish my story.

Paul Hausch

Fred Shull, M.D.
1415 Lakeway Dr.
Bellingham, WA 98226
206-733-9361

My hip was hurting me more and more over a number of years. I went to my local hospital for an x-ray which showed severe hip degeneration. The radiologist who I knew well said, "Fred, you need a hip replacement. See Bill (an orthopedic surgeon) he'll fix you right up." I read in Health Freedom News an article by Dr. Faber about reconstruction therapy. I called him up and he said that he had success with hips recommended for artificial replacement both before and for those who had trouble after replacement.

I flew to Milwaukee and got my back and hip treated. Dr. Faber told me the back must also be treated in cases of hip problems. I got 4 vigorous treatments from him in 5 days, he then referred me to Dr. Koch in my state and I completed my therapy with him.

I have been able to roller skate and do artistic kite flying things I greatly enjoy in my retirement. I am allowing

(Turn to Page 213 before contacting these people.)

publication of this because I know from my many years of experience that artificial replacement parts and surgery often give less than the best results. If you call me for verification please leave your number. I'll return your call collect. I'm best found at home on weekends.

Fred Shull, M.D.
Graduate of Yale, Princeton
and State University of New York

CHRONIC FOOT PAIN

Albert A. Slang
1601 Riverdale Drive
Green Bay, Wis 54313
414-494-7995

For the last 15 years I've had aching, pain & soreness of both feet. At age 7 or 8 I cut my foot with an axe. I recovered from that. About 5 years ago I had poor movement of left big toe. I saw physician who found several spurs. He said, "I can live with it or have surgery." The foot pain made me feel that I had gout. I didn't but it sure hurt. I had to change my walk so that I turned my foot in so I didn't have to bend the big toe of the left foot. I preferred tennis shoes, just putting on dress shoes caused my toe to bend with high pain resulting. I had constant pain in my big toe.

I decided to live with it because bone surgery was not for me. I heard Dr. Faber's lecture in Manitowoc. It made sense. I also knew people that got better with his treatment. I decided to get the treatments. Right away I noticed more stability, less pain and could flex my great toe. My feet are

(Turn to Page 213 before contacting these people.)

altogether different. I can feel my feet are essentially new now.

Permission to publish.

Albert A. Slang

CHRONIC NECK AND HEADACHE PAIN

Pam Thorpe
532 Mount Vernon
Oshkosh, Wi 54901

Dr. Faber of the Milwaukee Pain Clinic suspected that I had an injection in my jaw bone and sent me to a special dentist, Dr. Spaeth. Dr. Spaeth scraped both the top and bottom of my jaw bone on the left hand side of my mouth.

The next day, I noticed my neck was looser and the tightness on the left side of my neck disappeared. I also felt a little more mental clarity. I felt better all over and I can tell my fatigue will be better after all my dental work is done.

Pam Thorpe

Gena Henderson
2730 N. 46th St.
Milwaukee, Wi 53210
414-444-3500

Dear Milwaukee Observer,

I happened to see the program on RECONSTRUCTION THERAPY Saturday morning at 6:30. I found the program very interesting and want to thank you for the service you

(Turn to Page 213 before contacting these people.)

are doing in making this non-surgical treatment available - I had no idea such things were possible! Even though my background is in physical therapy (20 yrs. ago!) these treatments were not being used then. The research articles and testimonials were extremely interesting to me.

Sincerely,

Gena Henderson

CHRONIC NECK, BACK AND HIP PAIN

Betty Lou Thompson
1120 S. 120th St.
West Allis, Wi 53214
258-7480

For about 10-12 years, I have had pain in my lower back which caused me to see a Chiropractor. Then, about 6 years ago, my neck started to give me problems related to a fall off a horse as a teenager. In college, I had what appeared to be a little paralysis in my right hip and leg, which lasted for a couple of months. At that time, I did not seek any medical help. As the years went my pelvis and hip would always go out of joint.

I had a friend who attended a Barley Green meeting and heard Dr. Faber speak at the meeting. I decided to call him and make an appointment. I was very apprehensive about having the injections, but I had to have some relief from the pain. I started the injection therapy and was amazed that by the second treatment the results were remarkable. My hip feels firmer and stronger all the time.

The Milwaukee Pain Clinic is like a gift from God. I'm extremely happy with the results.

I'd be so happy to talk to anyone about my treatments at the Milwaukee Pain Clinic. It is too bad more people could not be aware of the benefits that result from Dr. Faber's treatments.

You may publish my story.

Betty Thompson

SCOLIOSIS, CHRONIC BACK AND HIP PAIN

William Bernatz
2467 S. 8th St.
Milwaukee, Wi 53215
383-2191

About 7 years ago, I developed a pain in my right hip, I had no appetite, I could not sleep. I could not work and I was in constant pain.

I went to a doctor and they told me to have some colonic treatment which I did. This loosened the pain in the lower back but the treatment took some of the pain away for only one day. I then found another doctor and I had an hour massage every 2 weeks but that was temporary relief also. I then went to another doctor and he gave me some adjustments with very little relief.

After a stand up X-ray another doctor decided I needed a lift in my shoe. He said the problem was that I was walking crooked with one shoulder higher than the other. I tried the lift and while it did help there was not that much difference in the pain. I then had a bone scan and an X-ray by an Orthopedic doctor and was told that they could find nothing wrong with my back.

I called the Milwaukee Pain Clinic and I started the Injection Therapy offered by the Milwaukee Pain Clinic. After a short period of the injection therapy, I eliminated the lift in my shoe and I have no more pain. I have had permanent relief for my back pain.

I do believe the Milwaukee Pain Clinic does a wonderful job in the relief of pain and I am very satisfied with the results.

I have recommended the Milwaukee Pain Clinic to many of my friends and I will be happy to discuss my treatments with anyone that contacts me.

You may publish my story.

William Bernatz

INSTANT RELIEF OF CHRONIC BACK PAIN

Charles Krueger
W6764 Hy 10
Appleton, Wi 54915
1-757-5158

For 3 years I had pain between the shoulder blades (Thorasic area) due to a broken back that fused itself about 18 years ago.

I went to two Orthopedic surgeons, had nerve blocks done, went through therapy and then went to a Neurosurgeon and he suggested surgery. I had a laminectomy and a Sensory Neurectomy in 1989. I was pain free for about 6 months.

The pain returned and I went through therapy again and September of 1990 they put a Tens Unit on me. This helped so I could move slowly, but did not really take care of the pain. I didn't know what to do anymore and just by luck, I got a hold of Dr. Faber's book Pain, Pain Go Away. I read the book and decided to call for an appointment.

I started the Neural Therapy and got immediate relief. I got up off the table with no pain. The car ride to my home did

(Turn to Page 213 before contacting these people.)

not bother me.

I think the Milwaukee Pain Clinic is super excellent. Dr. Faber is the answer to my prayers. It feels so good to be pain free. I don't know how to act.

I certainly will talk to anyone that call about my treatments that made me pain free.

You may publish my story.

Charles Krueger

Kathleen Maxson
W278 S3206 Marlene Ln.
Waukesha, Wi 53188
968-2288

I have had headaches for years but the last 2 years they got progressively worse, and I had daily headaches. I woke up every morning with one.

I had been to several doctors and they put me on medication. Another doctor put me on a muscle relaxer and told me I had an arthritic neck. I was told to live with the pain. I didn't want to live with the pain any longer because I had been living with the pain. I was then put on Hormone Therapy and that did not help. My dentist then took X-rays, thinking the pain was from TMJ.

I listened to Dr. Faber of the Milwaukee Pain Clinic on W.T.M.J. and ordered the book. I decided to try the injection therapy and called the Milwaukee Pain Clinic for appointment.

Dr. Faber recommended I go to see a special dentist, which I did and had my widom teeth pulled out. I had very serious fatigue and thought it was from taking so many pain pills. My fatigue was better after the teeth were pulled out.

Dr. Faber started the injection therapy and I noticed the

(Turn to Page 213 before contacting these people.)

headache was not as severe and as frequent. My neck now feels firmer and the headaches are getting better all the time.

I do believe I have found my answer at the Milwaukee Pain Clinic.

I have many friends that are interested in talking to me about my treatment at the Clinic.

You may publish my story.

Kathleen Maxson

TOE AND ABDOMINAL PAIN

Sylvia Woods
3626 E. Holmes Avenue
Cudahy, WI 53110
(414) 481-1210

I had surgery in 1948 for my appendix and a cyst. The scar gave me such a pulling sensation and it made me feel sick to touch it. I had been to see a chiropractor and orthopedic doctors. Their advice was to learn to live with the pain.

I saw Dr. Faber on Channel 30 and I thought he could help me so I called for an appointment. I came to the Milwaukee Pain Clinic and started the injection therapy and I immediately responded to the treatment in a positive way.

I can now move my toes on my left foot and I was not able to do that for years. I felt lighter and the pain from my hip to the mid back has disappeared. The sensation in my scar is less and I'm feeling better.

The Milwaukee Pain Clinic has restored my desire to live. I would gladly discuss my treatment at the clinic with anyone. You may publish my story.

Sylvia Woods

(Turn to Page 213 before contacting these people.)

TWO FAILED BACK SURGERIES

Mark Myszewski
4408 s. 5th Place
Milwaukee, WI 53207

I have had pain in my left leg, plus a dull numbing pain in my back since August of 1990 from moving some furniture.

Prior to this, I had a laminectomy in February of 1989. Following that my leg and back started to hurt again so I went back to the doctor who had done the laminectomy. I had an MRI and I found that the disc had herniated again. The doctor suggested I have surgery again so I had another laminectomy in January of 1991. I had no relief from the pain following this second surgery. I had leg and back pain continuously.

My parents saw Dr. Faber on Channel 30 and we made an appointment to see him. I wanted relief from the pain so I started the injection therapy.

I had almost instantaneous relief and I am pain free. I think the Milwaukee Pain Clinic is a great place to come for anyone in pain or disability.

I will gladly discuss my treatments and tell anyone else in pain to (go for it). You may publish my story.

Mark Myszewski

(Turn to Page 213 before contacting these people.)

FAILED BACK SURGERY

Richard Neff
2904 S. 19th St
Manitowoc, WI 54220
682-4806

In July, 1979 I slipped at work and when I tried to catch myself I injured my back. I sought medical help and the doctor gave me B12 shots. I developed such back pain I could not move my legs. At this time I was given heat treatments but they did not help . I was then advised to see an orthopedic doctor and he put me in traction for several days. He then suggested an exercise program and medication. The orthopedic doctor then suggested I have a myelogram and recommended surgery on my back.

I did not want the surgery but the company I worked for told me I would have to have the surgery because if I did not I would not be covered by the medical insurance in the future. I did go ahead and had a laminectomy on my low back.

I kept having pain and when I went back to the doctor he gave me more pain pills and valium. I again injured my back by slipping on the loading dock. I had another myelogram and the doctor prescribed pain medication. I got very ill, throwing up, and had a numb feeling in my back.

A friend had been to see Dr. Faber at the Milwaukee Pain Clinic and had gotten relief from pain so I decided to call Dr. Faber and make an appointment.

I started the injection therapy and got almost immediate relief and I no longer have the terrible spasms in my back. I think the Milwaukee Pain Clinic is absolutely terrific and

(Turn to Page 213 before contacting these people.)

unbelievable. I'm so happy with the results.

Anyone may call me at any time and I will discuss my treatments and tell them how strong and firm my back feels. You may publish my story.

Richard Neff

CHRONIC LOW BACK PAIN

James Donald Wanless
Route 5 Box 650
Richland Center, WI 53581

In 1954 at the age of 13 I was thrown off a tractor and landed on my feet. It felt like I was "crushed together." I have had pain ever since.

From time to time I looked for some medical help and I saw some chiropractors. They did not feel there was anything they could do for me.

I heard Dr. Faber, of the Milwaukee Pain Clinic, present a seminar at the Brewer Science Library Foundation, of which I am the President of the Board of Directors. So, I decided to call for an appointment to see if Dr. Faber could help the pain.

When I came to Dr. Faber's office, he sent me for X-rays and it was discovered that I had an infection in my jaw bone. Dr. Faber sent me to a special denstist and he scraped my jaw bone.

I then started the injection therapy and I had almost immediate relief. I could just tell my back felt better after the first treatment.

What a relief to find a place like the Milwaukee Pain Clinic which is geared to using a non-drug treatment, rather than being given a prescription for pain pills, which is what

(Turn to Page 213 before contacting these people.)

most other doctors do.

I will certainly talk to anyone about my treatments at the clinic and have already told many of my friends. You certainly may publish my story.

HIP PAIN AND HEEL SPURS

Larry Krak
Box 145
Gilman, WI 54433
(715) 447-5739

I have had a pain in my hip from an injury in 1965 when I ran into a brick wall playing hardball. The X-ray showed I had arthritis deterioration.

I went to a doctor and he suggested I have a hip replacement. I wanted no part of that. I heard Dr. Faber of the Milwaukee Pain Clinic speak on Wisconsin Public Radio and I sent for his book, Pain, Pain Go Away. I read the book and decided to call for an appointment.

I started the injection therapy on my hip and on some bone spurs in my heel. I noticed some marked relief after my first treatment and as I continue treatments my pain is almost gone.

The Milwaukee Pain Clinic is a very fine facility. The way your questions are answered is terrific, the waiting rooms are very nice and all the people are so friendly. The clinic is an easy place to find.

I will be happy to discuss my treatments at the Milwaukee Pain Clinic with anyone that calls me.

You may publish my story.

(Turn to Page 213 before contacting these people.)

BIRTH TRAUMA WITH CRANIAL DEFORMITY

Greg Weber
N8689 County Trunk W
Malone, WI 53049
(414) 795-4068

Greg was born September 11, 1986 in the city of Fond du Lac. When I was having Gregory I was probably in labor for six hours. When it was time for him to be born the nurse was pushing on my stomach and Greg was coming out. His head was out just for a minute and all of a sudden he was gone. He went back through the birth canal. They had to work on pushing on my stomach all over again until he was born. So Greg went through my birth canal two times.

When he was about 2 years old my babysitter noticed how his one eye was off to the side (left eye). I took him in to my doctor and he sent me to the eye doctor. The eye doctor didn't seem to think there was anything wrong. He thought the bone in his nose would grow and then the skin would lift up and he wouldn't have any problems. This was in Septemeber of 1988. The eye doctor told me to bring him back before he started school so we didn't do anything else until we came down to see Dr. Faber in November 1990.

My mom was down here getting help from Dr. Faber and Gregory and I brought her down. Greg and I went into the room with her and Dr. Faber was interested in why Greg's eye was off. He asked if I had been on any drugs during the pregnancy which I was not.

I brought my husband to Dr. Faber and he was explaining what was wrong with Gregory — how narrow his head was and how his eye was off and how this may be affecting his behavior. So we started treatment on him in November, 1990.

Greg's behavior is better in the following ways. There are days he now sits lots longer and looks at books. He loves for

(Turn to Page 213 before contacting these people.)

you to read to him and then he starts to read it. So, now in February his eyes are starting to drain and Dr. Faber says this is a good sign. Everyone notices how much better Greg's head looks. Greg's eyes are now normal.

The people are really friendly to us and Greg is such a celebrity down here everybody knows him and loves him. I really appreciate that. Yes, you may publish this.

LOST EYESIGHT — INSTANT IMPROVEMENT

Anne Fleming
508 - 1480m Foster St.
White Rock, B.C. CANADA Y4B3Y7

On May 19, 1981 I was walking down the street and as I got to the corner I fell and hit the curb with my right eye. Immediately my eye "popped out" with a goose egg so I was taken to the hospital. They took me to the emergency room where they checked my right shoulder and told me there was no evidence of a fracture and sent me home. The doctor asked me if I could see double and I said, "No." In fact, I could not see anything out of my eye.

My husband called a friend, an optometrist, and that doctor sent me to an opthamologist immediately. He examined me and said, "You have torn an optic nerve and you will not get your sight back."

I then went to see a neurologist and this doctor took X-rays and said, "I'm sorry this is tragic and serious. This is only the 3rd case I've seen like this and I suggest you learn to live with it."

I then tried cranial therapy, acupuncture, physical therapy and supplements but nothing helped.

Since my hip had gotten worse I heard about a doctor in Washington and I made an appointment to see him. He

(Turn to Page 213 before contacting these people.)

examined my hip and suggested surgery. We then got notice that Dr. Faber of the Milwaukee Pain Clinic would be attending the Canadian Consumer Health Convention as a speaker. We decided to attend the meeting. We attended the meeting and attempted to talk to Dr. Faber but there were so many people crowded around him we couldn't see him. At this point we decided to call for an appointment.

Dr. Faber asked questions about my eye and he stated he would try to help my eye. This gave me some hope because long ago I had given up hope.

I started the injection therapy on the eye and after the first treatment, the dark gray appearing curtain over the eye got lighter and I noticed a white light line at the bottom of the eye. After the 2nd treatment the dark curtain got a little lighter again. After the 3rd treatment the curtain keeps getting lighter and there is less cloudiness now.

I am very optimistic about the treatments on my eye and I have so much faith in Dr. Faber. I will gladly discuss my treatments with anyone that contacts me.

You may publish my story.

Anne Fleming

(Turn to Page 213 before contacting these people.)

AFTERWORD

Our authorship of this book is a starting place for bringing the advanced science of neural/fascial therapy to the medical consumer in easy to understand language. It is not meant to be encyclopedic in nature, but rather an introduction to the basic concepts of neural/fascial treatment.

Authors wish to cover their subjects comprehensively; therefore, we are planning to accomplish such coverage in a series of books. The next one—our third—to be called Goodby Back and Hip Pain, which will be followed by the fourth—Goodby Head and Neck Pain. Other books, booklets, and audiovisual projects are planned as well. Life is too short to live it with pain and disability, and our goal is to continue with researching, practicing, writing, teaching, lecturing, and producing communications so that others can permanently end their suffering.

—William J. Faber, D.O.
and
Morton Walker, D.P.M

APPENDIX I

WORLD DOCTORS WHO ADMINISTER NEURAL/FASCIAL THERAPY

...Before you consult the listed doctors for neural/fascial therapy —

Neural/fascial therapy is both an art and science. It's effectiveness is dependent upon the understanding and experience of the treating physician. These skills are not universal nor are they equal among practitioners of Neural/fascial therapy. The authors and publisher do not accept any responsibility for the professional activities of the physicians listed. One neural/fascial therapist may not get results while another with more experience and understanding will. The scope of neural/facial therapy is not to be construed as injection of scars. Dr. Hopfer of Austria states that only a small portion of neural therapy is scars. Neural therapy encompasses all of clinical anesthesia and far more. This is not to say that a certified anesthesiologist knows neural therapy concepts and performs neural/fascial therapy. Unfortunately there is a critical need for more physicians to learn these broadened concepts.

Be leery of the physician who uses cortisone and its similars. Cortisone is not compatible with the self-regulation principles of neural therapy.

The authors believe neural/fascial therapy properly applied is an effective and wonderful treatment for many who have not been able to find relief with other methods. The material here is not the practice of medicine and should not be considered such. The material here is factual and is considered educational in nature. Those seeking health advice and treatment are directed to select the health practitioner of their choice.

Those wishing an updated list of practitioners and other correspondence please send a self addressed stamped envelope to, Dr. Faber. He will add physicians to the list as he trains them. Physicians wishing to be added to the list without Dr. Faber's training, must demonstrate their specific training and experience to his satisfaction.

Dr. Faber will not endorse any physician's skills so please don't request comments about same. Neural/fascial therapy is both a science and an art, and as in life there are no guarantees given or implied.

Ausländische Mitglieder

Dr. med.
Göbel, Johannes
D-8562 Hersbruck
Breslauer Str. 19
Dr. med.
Kirchlechner, Othmar
Verdistr. 5
I-39012 Meran / Italien

Dr. med.
Turek, Paul
S-62100 Visby/Gotland
Schweden

ARGENTINA

Dr. med.
Schreiber, Marco Fco.
Malabrigo (Santa Fe)

AUSTRALIA

Dr. med.
Stoijc, Bogdan
42 Centr. A. Beauty P.
2088 N.S.W., Sydney

AUSTRIA

Dr. med.
Göbel, Johannes
D-8563 Hersbruck
Breslauer Str. 19

Dr. med.
Kirchlechner, Othmar
Verdistr. 5
I-39012 Meran / Italien

Dr. med.
Turek, Paul
S-62100 Visby/Gotland
Schweden

BELGIUM

Dr. med.
Adam, Andre
Prins Albertlei 7
B-2600 Berchem

Dr. med.
Bauwens, Maurice
Dennenstrast 14
B-3260 Bekkevooort

Dr. med.
Debeuckelaere, M.
Stat. Straat 17, Bus 4
B-9300 Aals

Dr. med.
Beer, A. D.E.
Zuidstraat 55
B-8800 Roeselare

Dr. med.
van Belle Laurent
Haneveldlaan 15
B-1850 Grimbergen

Dr. med
Bottu, Maurice
Beauduinstraat 143
B-3300 Tienen

Dr. med.
van Braeckel, J.
J. van Ophemstraat 16
B-3220 Aarschot

Dr. med.
van der Burgth, Paul
Dorpsstraat 147 G 18
B-9410 Erpe

Dr. med.
Buyle, Evelyn

Zoutelaan 176
B-8300 Knokke

Dr. med.
Campen, Dirk
Haaehtse Baan 102
B-2850 Keerbergen

Dr. med.
Daenen, J.
Mechelsesteenweg 163
B-2018 Antwerpen

Dr. med.
Degeling, Maria
20, Eug. Dierckxlaan
B-2230 Schilde

Dr. med.
Dejonghe, D.
De Robianostraat 2
B- 1980 Tervuren

Dr. med.
Diels, Alfons
Leeks 59
B-2440 Geel

Dr. med.
Dousselaere-Follet
G. Martensstraat 14
B-9800 Deinze

Dr. med.
van Drogenbroek, Mich.
Kapelstraat 53
B-2890 Schriek

Dr. med.
Fobelets
Tiensestraat 19
B-3451 Kortenaken

Dr. med.
Godderis, J.

St. Donaastraat 1
B-8380 Zeebrugge

Dr. med.
van Gronsveld, Frans
Steenweg
B-3771 Riemst

Dr. med.
De Kerpel, Jan
Denderhoutenbaan 116
B-9400 Ninove

Dr. med.
Leysen, Paul
Dorpstraat
B-2170 Wuustwezel

Dr. med.
Lombaerts, Frans
Waterlolaan 92
B-1020 Brüssel

Dr. med.
Maertens, C
Buissetstraat 37
B-1800 Vilvoorde

Dr. med.
de Mayer, W.
Rucaplein 552
B-2610 Wilrijk

Dr. med.
Mertens, Ferdinand
Steenw. op Nieuwr. 35
B-3111 Wezemaal

Dr. med.
Mertens, Jules
Aarschotsesteen 126
B-3111 Rotselaar

Dr. med.
Mommeyer, K.

Engstegenseweg 2
B-3520 Zonhoven

Dr. med.
Nuyens, Michel
Hofkwartier 5
B-2410 Herentals

Dr. med.
van Orshoven
Heymanswef 3
B-3694 Neerglabbeek

Dr. med.
Otten, Philip
K. V. Overmeirelaan 4
B-2100 Deurne

Dr. med.
Otten, Philip
K.V. Overmeirenlaan 4
B-2100 Deurne

Dr. med.
Paesmaas, M.
Kanaalstraat 7
B-3582 Neerpelt

Dr. med.
Rathe, Etienne
Brusselbaan 82 A
B-1790 Hekelgem

Dr. med.
Rinchart, R.
Av. de Broquev. 272/13
B-1150 Brüssel

Dr. med.
Roovers, Serge
Eeekhoornlaan 41
B-2610 Wilrijk

Dr. med.
van Roy, G.
Sociale Straat 6
B-3600 Genk

Dr. med.
Schellens, Ludo
Schrunmarkers-Str. 19
B-3000 Leuven

Dr. med.
Slachmuylders, J.
Maantjessteenweg 65
B-2060 Merksem

Dr. med.
Timmermans, Liesbeth
J. Sermonlaan 10
B-1080 Ganshoren

Dr. med.
Verhaert, Louis
Liersebaan 8
B-2550 Kontich

Dr. med.
Verbruggen
Aardbeziestraat
B-3990 Meerhout

Dr. med.
Verroken, Bartel
Beverstraat 62
B-9700 Qudenaarde

Dr. med.
Weynants, H.
Statiestraat 123
B-2730 Zwijndrecht

Dr. med.
Wouters, J.
Eikenstraat 94

BULGARIA

Dr. med. dent.
Bossner, Iwan
Boul. Stamoliiski 22
Sofia
Zahnarzt

Dr. med.
Bossnew, W.
Boul. Stamoliiski 22
Sofia
Neurologe

Dr. med.
Goscheff, Dimiter
Ul. Sofronie 16
Sofia III
Internist

CANADA

Jean Aubry MD
65 B Queen
PO Box 2230
Sturgeon Falls Ontario POH 2G0

Indra Deepan MD
226 Sydney Street
Cornwall Ontario K6H 3H4

Werner Fabian MD
5 Robert Street
Thornton Ontario LOL 2N0

John Hopkins MD
64 Bridle Path
Don Mills Ontario

Lionel Labbé MD
204-260 Dalhousie
Ottawa Ontario KIN 7E4

Oscar Lee MD
800 Bathurst St.
Suite 207
Toronto Ontario M5R 3M8

Dr. med.
Bajusz, Eoers
University of Montreal
Montreal

COLUMBIA

(Südamerikanische Gesellschaft)
siehe III

CZECHOSLOVAKIA

MUDR. M. Beno, M.
Hviezdoslavova 6
CS-96232

Doz. Dr.
Lezovic, Jan
Bezrucova 5
Bratislava

Dr. MED.
Salansky, Igor
Ponavka 6
Brno

EGYPT

Dr. med.
Hosny, Abbas
Rue Hasr el Nil
Kairo

FINLAND

Dr. med.
Krohn, Kari
Haemeentatu 21 C 46
15110 Lahti

FRANCE

Dr. med.
Bach, Carl
3, Rue Theodore Deck
F-67000 Strassburg
Homöopathie

Dr. med.
Cucheval, Luc
Pas de Calais
Colembert

Dr. med.
de Kuyper, Philippe
6, Rue de Let. de Tass
F-78000 Versailles

Dr. med.
Pelz, Gonthier
49 Boulevard Pereire
F-75017 Paris

Dr. med.
Pierre Lous Richand
32, Avenue C. Mandel
F-75116 Paris

Dr. med.
Warter, Arcadius
36, Allee des Soundanes
F-78430 Louveciennes

Dr. med.
Weill, Elie
Vogesenstr. 26
F-67000 Strassburg

GERMANY

Dr. med.
Abele, Adold
F. — Ebert-Str. 40 1/10
6090 Rüsselsheim
Tel.: 06142/65114
Gynäkologe

Dr. med.
Adjodani, Bahram
Gruner Weg 6
4100 Duisburg — 46
Tel.: 0203/409686
Allgemeinmed.

Dr. med.
Al-Bayati, K.
Bahnhofstr. 16
4050 Mönchegladbach

Dr. med.
Albrecht, Rudolf
Cosimastr. 224
8000 München — 81
Tel.: 089/951535
Allgemeinmed.

Dr. med.
Albus, Tassilo
Kathreinerstr 26
8939 Bad Wörishofen
Tel. 08247/5626

Dr. med.
Andrews, Helmut
Spielberg 5
7997 Immenstadt
Tel.: 07543/6808
Internist

Dr. med.
Angerer, Liselotte
Heubergstr. 36
8229 Mitterfelden

Dr. med.
Armbrüster. Alfred
Unterm Heilgkreuz 9

6400 Fulda
Tel.: 0661/73040
Internist

Dr. med.
Artmann, Michael
Ludwigstr. 1
8070 Ingolstadt

Dr. med.
Auch, Erich
Haupstr. 98
7831 Eichstetten a. K.
Tel.: 07663/2041
Allgemeinmed.

Dr. med.
Augustin, Hans-Peter
Hauptstr. 307
4133 Neukirchen-Vluyn
Tel.: 02845/2362
Allgemeinmed.

Dr. med.
Baecker, Karl
Am Schützenhof 7
2390 Flensburg
Tel.: 0461/51105
Allgemeinmed.

Dr. med.
Balaban, Romulus
Postfach 1120
3256 Coppenbrügge 1

Dr. med.
Banani, Cyrus
Kurfürstendamm 97-98
1000 Berlin — 31
Tel.: 030/3234049
Allgemeinmed.

Dr. med.
Bark, Christian
Gartenfelder Str. 86
1000 Berlin — 20
Tel.: 030/3344954

Dr. med.
Barop
Hostenstr. 2
2000 Hamburg — 50

Dr. med.
Baumgart, Charlotte
Gerichtsstr. 30
4937 Lage/Lippe

Dr. med.
Bausch, Michael
Kronenstr. 15
7400 Tübingen

Dr. med.
Bay, Tilman
K. — Adenauer-Str. 13
7208 Spaichingen
Tel.: 07424/7100
Allgemeinmed.

Dr. med.
Beck, Jörg
Tannenweg 23
8858 Neubury-Ried
Tel.: 08431/44222

Dr. med.
Becker, H.-J.
Jasperallee 5
3300 Braunschweig
Tel.: 0531/338357
Zahnarzt

Dr. med.
Behrmann, Wolfgang
Horststr. 35
2210 Oelixdorf

Dr. med
Bennemann, Jürgen
Kopmanshof 75
3250 Hameln-1

Dr. med.
Bercher, E.
Rittnerstr. 82
7500 Karlsruhe — 41

Dr. med.
Berger, Hugo
Ostpreussenstr. 6
6109 Mühltal — 3
Tel.: 06151/5933105

Dr. med.
Berghoff, Dieter
Hindenburgstr. 34
2060 Bad Oldesloe

Dr. med.
Berkhoff, Gerhard
Rennweg 7
4722 Bad Sassendorf

Dr. med.
Beyer, Harald
2421 Hutzfeld/Eutin
Tel.: 04527/206
Allgemeinmed.

Dr. med.
Birk, Walter
3569 Altenvers
Tel.: 06426/886
Allgemeinmed.

Dr. med.
Bischoff, Fr.-G.
Wilhelmstr. 26-28
4970 Bad Oeynhausen
Tel.: 05731/20549 + 20288
Internist

Dr. med.
Blessing, Hugo
7959 Obersulmettingen 42
Tel.: 07392/3476
Allgemeinmed.

Dr. med.
Blome, Götz
Hildastr. 59
7800 Freiburg
Tel.: 0761/73455
Naturheilverf.

Dr. med.
von Blumenthal, R
Pestalozzistr. 18
6953 Gundelsheim
Tel.: 06269/363
Allgemeinmed.
Naturheilverf.

Dr. med.
Böhm, Käthe
Stadtwald 16
6300 Giessen/Lahn
Tel.: 0641/43241
Allgemeinmed.

Dr. med.
Böhm, Udo
Haupstr. 64
8218 Unterwössen
Allgemeinmed.

Dr. med.
Bommer, Justinus
Asternweg 5
7253 Renningen-Malmsheim
Tel.: 07159/2624
Allgemeinmed.

Dr. med.
Bönig, Rita
Hohe Brücke

4052 Korschenbroich

Dr. med.
Baonnemann, Detlef
Detmolder Str. 419
4800 Bielefeld — 1

Dr. med.
Both, Lucia
Quendtstedter Str. 30 A 27
7400 Tübiingen

Dr. med.
Braemer, Christel
Bitterstr. 24
1000 Berlin-Dahlem
Tel.: 030/8312437
Homöopathie

Dr. med.
Brammer, Helmut
Maschstr. 18
2840 Diepholz

Dr. med.
Brandt, Walter
Birkenweg 12
8501 Schwaig b. Nürnberg
Tel.: 0911/574340
Allgemeinmed.

Dr. med.
Braun, Helmut
In den Weiden 17
Tel.: 06842/51491
Internist

Dr. med.
Bretschneider Fritz
Hönnetalstr. 34
5872 Deilinghofen
Tel.: 02372/6704
Allgemeinmed.

Dr. med.
Britz, Erhard
Neuer Weg 26
5450 Neuwied 13
Naturheilverf.

Dr. med.
Brückmann, Walter
Adalbertstr. 37
2300 Kiel 1
Tel.: 0431/336140
Gynäkologe

Dr. med.
Brügelmann, Hanns
Hartenthalerstr. 29
8939 Bad Wörishofen

Dr. med.
Brüning, E.
SchloBstr. 4
4408 Dülmen
Tel.: 02594/5045
Allgemeinmed.

Dr. med.
Buchhheit, Hubertus
Alte Markstr. 1
6653 Bleiskastel
Tel.: 06842/2504
Gynäkologe

Dr. med.
Bürger, Horst D.
8906 Gerstenhofen/Augsbg.
Tel. 0821/491080
Zellulartherapie

Dr. med.
Bürger, Josef
Am Himmelsberg 2
7912 Weissenhorn-Wallenhs.
Tel.: 07309/2455
Algemeinmed.

Dr. med.
Büttner, Peter-Gerd
Erlenweg12
8192 Geretsried

Dr. med. Privatdozent
Burmeister, Hannelore
Badstr. 67
1000 Berlin — 65

Dr. med.
Buschmann. S.
Am. Hünensteinn 12
2860 Osterholz-Scharmbeck

Dr. med
Cantner, Christine
Waldstr. 12
6990 Bad Mergentheim
Naturheilverf.

Dr. med.
Colombo, Ralph-Th.
Fuggerstr. 36
8930 Schwabmünchen
Tel.: 08232/4424
Allgemeinmed.

Dr. med.
Conrad, Albert
Ritter-Simon-Weg 6
5220 Waldbröl
Tel. 02291/3030
Allgemeinmed.

Dr. med.
Cosentino, Magda
Fredericiastr. 16
1000 Berlin — 19

Dr. med.
Dallmann, Peter
Kniebisstr. 7
7291 Sweewald-Besenfeld
Tel.: 07448-300
Allgemeinmed.
Dr. med.
Dankwardt, Renate
Bauernvogtkopp. 27 b
2000 Hamburg — 65
Tel.: 040/6014610
Allgemeinmed.

Dr. med.
Darkoh, Godfried-S.-
Herderstr. 6
3280 Bad Pyrmont
Allgemeinmed.
Anästhesie

Daske, Klaus
Steinberger Str. 17
7901 illerstrieden-Dorndorf
Zahnarzt

Dr. med.
Daxl, Jürgen
Freisinger Str. 14
8302 Mainburg
Tel.: 08751/1338
Allgemeinmed.

Dr. med.
Dichter, Karl-Heinz
Herzogstr. 7
5100 Aachen
Tel.: 0241/505416
Allgemeinmed.

Dr. med.
Diedrichs, Klaus
Bahnhofstr. 13
6640 Merzing/Sarr
Tel.: 06688/2554
Allgemeinmed.

Dr. med.
Diehl, Wilhelm
Innere Münchner Str. 25
8300 Landshut
Tel.: 0871-3949
FA f. Orthopädie

Dr. med.

Djimjadi, Joseph
Am Stefananger 23
8904 Friedberg
Allgemeinmed.

Dr. med.
Doerfler, Julius
Am Rathenaupart 5
2000 Hamburg — 50
Tel.: 040/8801680
Internist

Dr. med.
Dörr, Helmut
K.-Wilhelm-Str. 15
6700 Ludwigshafen
Tel.: 0621/514493

Dr. med.
Doll. Wilhelm
Heinrichstr. 7
4690 Herne
Tel.: 02323/50773
Allgemeinmed.
Zahnarzt

Dr. med.
Dorstewlitz, Hartmut
Wasserburger Str. 37
8011 Kirchseeon
Tel.: 08091/2200
Allgemeinmed.

Dr. med.
Dosch, Mathias
Bertelestr. 68
8000 München — 71/Solln
Tel.: 089/7914678
Allgemeinmed.

Dr. med.
Dosch, Tobias
Dahmengraben 9
5100 Aachen
Tel.: 0241/28232

Dr. med.
Draczynski, Gisela
Rurstr. 11
5000 Köln — 41

Dr. med.
Dreyer, Hermann
Poststr. 1
2723 Scheessel

Dr. med.
Druschky, Eberhard
Druschky-Klinik GmbH
6927 Bad Rappenau
Tel.: 07264/1088
Chefarzt

Dr. med.
Ebert, Jende
Herdweg 43
7000 Stuttgart — 1

Dr. med.
Eckert, Peter
Gartenstr. 7
6331 Hohenahr/Erda
Tel.: 06446/535
Internist

Dr. med.
Eder, Manfred
Klosterweg 8
8233 Anger

Dr. med.
Eichenlaub, Claus
Arnoldstr. 4
4000 Düsseldorf

Dr. med. Eickelmann, Rich. Wilh.
Kneippstr. 9
Bad Wörishofen
Tel.: 08247/4755
Leitender Arzt

d. Kurparksanat.

Dr. med.
Ellinger, Manfred
Hauptstr. 70
7620 Oberkirch
Tel.: 07802/2501
Allgemeinmed.

Dr. med.
Elsen, Heinz-G.
Brockmüllerstr. 11 a
5170 Jülich
Tel.: 02461/3368
Internist

Dr. med.
Eltze, Dietlind
K.-Kollwitz-Str. 4
5000 Köln — 50
Tel.: 0221/353935

Dr. med.
Emrich, Helmut
Bahnhofstr. 1
6702 Bad Dürkheim
Tel.: 06322/1995

Dr. med.
Engels, Jürgen
Rabenhorst 6
2000 Hamburg — 65
Tel.: 040/5362636
Allgemeinmed.
Homöopathie

Dr. med.
Epperlein, Horst
Andreasstr. 37
6520 Worms
Tel.: 06241/26336
Internist
Dr. med.
Erbe, Gisela
Zollernstr. 25
7460 Balingen
Tel. 07433/8711
Allgemeinmed.

Dr. med.
Erben, Luise
Schlagsdorfer Str. 6
2449 Petersdorf

Dr. med.
Faber, Gerhard
Bitzenstr. 25
6718 Grünstadt
Tel.: 06359/82800
Gynäkologe

Dr. med.
Farien, Irene
Kirchhofalle 31
2300 Kiel

Dr. med.
Feldhaus, Heinz-Wern. Dürerstr. 2
4446 Hörstel

Dr. med.
Fellmer, Karl-Ernst
R. — Strauss-Str. 28/I
8000 München — 80
Tel.: 089/472588
Internist

Dr. med.
Fichter, Helmut
Okenstr. 52
7800 Freiburg/Breisgau
Tel.: 0761/52931
Allgemeinmed.

Dr. med.
Fiege, Mechthild
Ebersbachhof
7611 Gutach

Dr. med.

Filser, Bernhard
Bismarckstr. 6
6750 Haiserslautern
Tel.: 0631/93144
Internist

Dr. med.
Fischer, Lisel
Waldparkstr. 28 b
6800 Mannheim
Allgemeinmed.

Dr. med.
Fischer, Wilhelm
Beulerweg 31
5982 Neuenrade
Tel.: 02394/62126
Allgemeinmed.
Dr. med.
Fleischer, Johann
Viersener Str. 6
5000 Köln — 60
Tel.: 0221/73 42 73
Allgemeinmed.
FA f. Urologie

Dr. med.
Fonk, Ingrid
Haydnstr. 2
8132 Tutzing
Tel.: 08158/2925

Dr. med.
Freise, Hans-Robert
Turnhallestr. 53
7290 Freudenstadt
Tel.: 07441/5222

Dr. med.
Freise, Sirgrid
Strassburger Str. 43
7290 Freudenstadt
Tel.: 07441/4446

Dr. med.
Freund, Horst-Dietmar
Heidebrinker Str. 7
1000 Berlin — 65
Tel.: 030/4928761

Dr. med.
Friedenberg, Erika
Eichelbergstr. 19
7500 Harlsruhe
Tel. 0721/574357

Dr. med.
Friedenberg, Peter
Eichelbergstr. 19
7500 Karlsruhe
Tel.: 0721/574357

Dr. med.
Friedrichsen, Hans-P.
Theod. Storm-Allee 25
2082 Ütersen

Dr. med.
Fritzsche, Kurt
Charlottenstr. 3
6600 Saarbrücken — 1
Tel.: 0681/57356

Dr. med.
Frühauf, Hubert
Röhnstr. 80
6050 Offenbach
Tel.: 0611/853135
Allgemeinmed.
Naturheilverf.

Dr. med.
Fuch, Friedrich
Weisskirchnerstr. 24
8000 München — 71

Dr. med.
Gaertner, Wolfram
Possartstr. 29

8000 München — 80
Tel.: 089/400454
HNO-Facharzt

Dr. med.
Galla, Jürgen
Oderweg 5
6907 Nussloch

Dr. med.
Ganghof, Georg
Schlopweg 12
3320 Salzgitter 51
Tel.: 05341/35061
Allgemeinmed.
FA f. Innere Krankh

Dr. med.
Garten, Hans
Ottostr. 17
5100 Aachen

Dr. med.
Gauri, Hailash-K.
Uke Augenklinik
2000 Hamburg — 20

Dr. med.
Geiger, Detlef
Heilbronner Str. 10
7143 Vaihingen/Enz
Tel.: 07042/14433
Orthopädie —
Chirotherapie

Dr. med.
Geisinger Karl
H. — Fischer-Str. 52
7710 Donaueschingen
Tel.: 0771/3295

Dr. med.
Geiss, Friedrich
Blütenstr. 8a

8500 Nürnberg
Tel.: 0911/573438
Allgemeinmed.

Dr. med.
Gellhaus, Elisbeth
Caspar-Heinr.-SStr. 18
3490 Bad Driburg

Dr. med.
Gerhardt, Marcel
7983 Wilhelmsdorf
Tel. 07503/584

Dr. med.
Gerke, Peter
Bonnestr. 2
2126 Adendorf
Tel.: 04131/18112
Allgemeinmed.

Dr. med.
von Gesell-Payer,
Andreas
Heinz-Fuchs-Str. 29
6900 Heidelberg
Tel.: 06221/35125

Dr. med.
Giannikos, Lambros
Kinkelstr. 18
5000 Köln — 41

Dr. med.
Geibel, Wilhelm
Am Krigermal 43
5600 Wuppertal — 23
Tel.: 020/611236
Allgemeinmed.

Dr. med.
Giesenbauer, Heinz
Hindenburgstr. 5
2800 Bremem-Lesum
Tel.: 0421/630101

Allgemeinmed.
Geburtshelfer

Geishoff, W.
Raiffeisenstr. 4
4060 Viersen-Boisheim
Tel.: 02162/55601
Zahnarzt

Dr. med.
Giustiniani, F.
Luisenstr. 1
7850 Lörrach
Psychiatrie
Neurologie
Ganzheitsmed.

Dr. med.
Gleditsch, Jochen
Traunreuter Str. 23
8000 München — 90
Tel.: 089/682675
HNO-Facharzt u.
Zahnarzt

Dr. med.
Glose, W.
Stoppelfeld 5
2000 Hamburg — 73
Internist
Naturheilverf.

Dr. med.
Göbel, Fritz
Frauenkopfstr. 38
7000 Stuttgart-Frauenkopf
Tel.: 0711/332601
Allgemeinmed.

Dr. med.
Göbel, Johannes
Breslauer Str. 19
8562 Hersbruck
Tel.: 09151/2651
Allgemeinmed.

Dr. me.
Gothe, K.
Aachener Str. 522
5000 Köln — 41
Tel.: 0221/493914

Dr. med.
Gothe, Manfred
Neusser Str. 174
5000 Köln — 60
Tel.: 0221/738806
Allgemeinmed.

Dr. med.
Gothardt, M.
Theodor-Heuss-Str. 7
6750 Kaiserslautern
Allgemeinmed.

Dr. med.
Gottschalk, Sabine
Mozartstr. 7
7403 Ammerbuch — 1

Dr. med. Graefe, Hermann
Quintusstr. 78
3030 Walsrode

Dr. med.
Gröff, Volker
Hunsrückstr. 50
3500 Kassel

Dr. med.
Gramse, Erwin
Podbielski-A. 31-33
1000 Berliin-Dahlem
Tel.: 030/8325680
Chirurg

Dr. med.
Gramse, Erwin
K.-Friedrich-Ring 32

6200 Wiesbaden
Tel.: 06121/304101
Allgemeinmed.

Dr. med.
Griese, Manfred
Johannisstr. 24
2390 Flensburg

Dr. med.
Criessinger, Karl
Oberachweg 6
8283 Rottach-Egern
Tel.: 08022/26544
spez. Neuraltherapie

Dr. med.
Grosser, Lisa
Kalkumer Str. 137
4000 Düsseldorf — 30
Tel.: 0211/422734
Allgemeinmed.

Dr. med.
Grossmann, Klaus
Gärtnereigasse 7
3008 Garbsen —
Tel.: 0537/73127
Allgemeinmed.

Dr. med.
Grube, Fredo-Otto
Zeppelinstr. 26
8520 Erlangen

Dr. med.
Grüger, Wolfgang
Arndstr. 6 A
4755 Holzwickede
Tel.: 02301/2000
Allgemeinmed.
Chirurg
Dr. med.
Grutschkowski, Edmund
Bahnhofstr. 24
7253 Renningen
Tel.: 07159/3117

Dr. med.
Günther, Ernst
Söckinger Str. 25
8130 Starnberg
Tel.: 08151/14536
spez. Neuralth.

Dr. med.
Guethenke, Rolf
Prekerstr. 50
4830 Gütheraloh — 1
Tel.: 05241/5211
Naturheilverf.

Dr. med.
Gutmann, Gottfried
Rennweg 7
4772 Bad Sassendorf
Tel.: 02921/52001

Dr. med. de haas, Wolfgang
Müllerstr. 60
1000 Berlin — 65
Tel.: 030/4516521
HNO-Facharzt

Dr. med.
Habermaier, H.
Kaiserstr. 34
5200 Sieburg
Tel.: 02241/64195
Orthopädie

Dr. med.
Hänisch, Rainer
Holbeinstr. 28
1000 Berlin — 45
Tel.: 0030/8336384
Neuraltherapie
Dr. med.
Härtling, Hans
Lindenstr. 1

8391 Kellberg

Dr. med.
Hahn, Mathias
Glienicker Str. 9
1000 Berlin — 9

Dr. med.
Hahn-Godeffroy
Fr.-Legan-Str. 2
2000 Hamburg — 55

Dr. med.
Hallermann, Wilhelm
Castroper Str. 36
4600 Dortmund-Mengede
Tel.: 0231/337373
HNO-Facharzt

Dr. med.
Hamadeh, Riyad
Berliner Str. 46
6831 Neuleßheim
Tel. 06290/31933
Internist

Dr. med.
Harms, Hajo
Prieser Strand 5
2300 Kiel — 17

Dr. med.
Hardin, Ingeborg
Mauerstr. 1
4000 Düsseldorf

Dr. med.
Hartmann, Rüdiger Eulenhof 11
2862 Worbswede-Hüttenb.
Orthopädie

Dr. med.
Hartmann, Wolfgang
Marienhölzungsweg 5
2390 Flensburg

Dr. med.
Hasinger, Marg.
Lipowskystr. 30
8000 München — 70
Tel.: 089/7 25 43 00
Allgemeinmed.
Homöopathie

Dr. med.
Hasper, Ursula
Mosebergstr. 1
3423 Bad Sachsa

Dr. med.
Hatam, M.
Loewenichstr. 17
8520 Erlangen

Dr. med.
Hausmann, Paul
Neebs-Allee 9
2930 Varel/0
Tel.: 04451/2277

Dr. med.
Hausner, W.
Pfarrstr. 9
8572 Auerbach

Dr. med.
Hausser Dietrich
Rotebühlplatz 11
7000 Stuttgart — 1

Dr. med.
Hausleiter, Renate
Josephstr. 4
8000 München — 40
Tel.: 089/2714040
Naturheilverf.

Dr. med.
Heitsch, Rolf

L.-Richter-Str. 61
4350 Recklinghausen
Tel.: 02361/57200
Allgemeinmed.

Dr. med.
Henne-Gerth, Marianne
Heimstr. 39
7900 Ulm
Tel.: 0731/23468
Homöopathie

Dr. med.
Henss Helmut
Sulingerstr. 20
4500 Osnabrück
Tel.: 9541/15430

Dr. med.
Herbert, Hermann
Fringsstr. 17
4040 Neuss/Rhein
Tel.: 02101/42437
Allgemeinmed.

Dr. med.
Hertlein, Marold
Heringer Str. 16
8991 Hergensweiler
Tel.: 08388/803
Allgemeinmed.

Dr. med.
Herzog, Helmut
Weissenburger Str. 1
2000 Hamburg — 70

Dr. med.
Herzog, Ulrich
Nikolausberg 56
3400 Göttingen
Dr. med.
Heupel, Paul Joachim
Wielandstr. 5
5900 Siegen

Dr. med.
Heyn, Detlev
Speckenstr. 176
2839 Siedenburg
Tel: 04272/744

Dr. med.
Hildmann, Karl
Heinestr. 2
6000 Frankfurt/Main
Tel.: 0611/552421
HNO-Facharzt

Dr. med.
Himmel, Andreas
Dahlienstr. 71
4150 Krefeld

Dr. med.
Himmel, Andreas
Rechtmurgstr. 20
7292 Baiersbronn-Obertal

Dr. med.
Hinkel, Magdalene
Max-Reger-Str. 2
4370 Marl

Dr. med.
Hinze, Eduard
Max-Planck-Str. 4
3011 Garbsen-Havelse
Tel.: 05137/77791
Allgemeinmed.

Dr. med.
Hoenge, Herbert
Acisweg 8
6490 Schlüchtern
Tel.: 0661/811
Gynäkologe

Dr. med.

Hönighaus, Heribert
Münsterstr. 18
4417 Altenberge
Tel.: 02505/2361
Allgemeinmed.

Dr. med
Hoffman, Detlev
Haunauer Str. 39
6360 Friedberg — 1
Tel.: 06031/3800
Allgemeinmed.

Dr. med.
Hoffmann, Walter
Landwehr 29
2000 Hamburg — 76
Tel. 040/252154
Neuro-Psychiatrie

Dr. med.
Hoffmann, Wolfgang
Glienicker Str. 9
1000 Berlin — 39

Dr. med.
Hofius, Kurt
Hagensalle 54
4100 Duisburg — 12

Dr. med.
Hofmeister, Martha
Kaiserstr. 76
7417 Pfullingen
Tel.: 07121/71014
HNO-Fachärztin

Dr. med.
Holena, Arno
Wald. Marktplatz 11
2080 Pinneberg

Dr. med.
Homeyer, Alfons
Schwarzwaldstr. 45
6800 Mannheim — 1
Tel.: 0621/825363
Orthopädie
Sportmedizin

Dr. med.
Hoppe, Elisabeth
Friedrichstr. 37
4790 Paderborn

Dr. med.
Hose, Harald
Fermerlingstr. 11
2000 Hamburg — 90
Tel.: 040/7906240

Dr. med.
Hradil, Georg
Haupstr. 218
5060 Bergisch-Gladbach — 2
Tel.: 02202/34619
Allgemeinmed.

Dr. med.
Hubach, Hilde
Nr. 222 A
6799 Pfeffelbach/Kusel
Tel.: 06384/267
Allgemeinmed.

Dr. med.
Hüllemann, R.
Tibarg 24
2000 Hamburg — 61
Tel.: 040/587727
Gynäkologe

Dr. med.
Hülse, Werner
Hemigkofer Str. 18
7993 Kressbronn
Tel.: 07543/6555
Allgemeinmed.

Dr. med.
Huneke, Hagen
Mauritiusstr. 47
4005 Meerbusch-Buderich

Dr. med.
Huneke, Holger
Erwin-v.-Witzleben-Str. 17
4000 Düsseldorf-Nord
Tel.: 0211/435583/435583
Internist

Dr. med.
Huneke, Jürgen
Am Müllerberg 24
4934 Bad Meinberg
Tel.: 05234/9618
Allgemeinmed.
stationäre Be-
handlungsmöglichk.

Dr. med.
Hurrelmann, Franz
Theodor-Storm-Str. 18
8400 Regensburg
Tel.: 0941-991150
Allgemeinmed.

Dr. med.
Ilg, L.
Zermatter Str. 19
2800 Bremen — 44

Dr. med.
Iliescu, Vasile-Stelian
Frauenstr. 17
8000 München —
Tel.: 089/296126
Orthopädie
Rheumatologe
Unfallarzt

Dr. med.
Imm, Horst
Akazienstr. 50
4000 Düsseldorf - 22
Tel.: 0211/451845
spez. Neuralth.

Dr. med.
Irmer, Gotthard
Derkerborn 6
5790 Brilon im Wald
Tel.: 02961/2336
Allgemeinmed.

Dr. med.
Irrgang, Rosemarie
Wittestr. 8
4800 Bielefeld — 12
Tel.: 0521/40096
Allgemeinmed.

Dr. med.
Jancke, Georg-Hermann
Verdistr. 11
4010 Hildeh
Tel.: 02103/51144
Allgemeinmed.

Jentjens, Hermann
Elberfelder Str. 55
5608 Radevormw. — Bergerhof
Tel.: 02195/1025

Dr. med.
Jentzsch-Schilla G.
Limescorso 9
6000 Frankfurt — 50
Tel.: 0611/579900
Fachärztin für
Kieferorthopädie

Dr. med.
Jung, Eugen
Bahnhofstr. 25
6791 Hermersberg
Tel.: 06333/2473
Allgemeinmed.

Dr. med.
Kafai, Huschang
Neckarweg 13a
4800 Bielefeld-11

Dr. med.
Kamper, Bernd
Birkwäldele 18a
7801 Wittnau

Dr. med.
Kampik, Bernhard
Bürgerreuther Str. 39
8580 Bayreuth

Dr. med.
Kannegiesser Gerda
Rittnerstr. 15
7500 Karlsruhe — 41

Dr. med.
Karsch, Johannes
Gutenbergstr. 1
7560 Gaggenau
Tel.: 07225/3418
Augenarzt

Dr. med.
Kaufmann, Claus
Rathausstr. 8
3490 Bad Driburg/Westf.
Tel.: 9/05253/2681

Dr. med.
Kayling, Wolfgang
Schmaleichertorstr. 7
3576 Rauschenberg

Dr. med.
Kayser, Volker
Arnoldstr. 42
2000 Hamburg — 50
Dr. med.
Kayser, Walter
Bamenolhlerstr. 228
5950 Finnentrop
Tel.: 02721/7223
Allgemeinmed.

Dr. med.
Kern, Berthold
Reinsburgstr. 35a
7000 Stuttgart — West
Tel.: 0711/616495
Internist

Dr. med.
Kess, Elhard
Veersser Str. 62
3110 Ülzen — 1
Tel.: 0581/19933
Orthopädie

Dr. med.
Kettmeyer
Am Müllerberg 31
4934 Horn-Bad Meinberg 2
Tel.: 05234/98851
Allgemeinmed.

Dr. med.
Keymer, Rolf
Hesshofstr. 9
5000 Köln — 91
Tel.: 0221/871239
Orthopädie

Dr. med.
Kieper, Volkhart
An der Bahn 4
2061 Sülfeld
Tel. 04537/7793
Allgemeinmed.
Akupunktur
Neuraltherapie

Dr. med.
Kirsch, Herta-
Marianne

Saemannstr. 14
8032 Lochham/München
Tel: 089/876311
Allgemeinmed.

Dr. med.
Klehr, Fritz
H.-Dunant-Str. 3
8450 Amberg/Opf.
Tel.: 09621/82116
Allgemeinmed.

Dr. med.
Kleinstoll, Diethelm
Hürth-Park-Theresienhöhe
5030 Hürth 1
Tel.: 02233/72576
Allgemeinmed.
Chirotherapie
Sportmedizin

Dr. med.
Klenk, Gerhard
Beilsteiner Weg 6a
6600Saarbrücken — 2
Chirurgie
Sportmedizin

Dr. med.
Klingebiel, E.
Talstr. 59
6784 Thaleischweiler
Tel.: 06334/212
Allgemeinmedzin

Dr. med.
Klink, F.
Gärtnergasse 64
2400 Lübeck
Dr. med.
Klink, Gerhard
Heinestr. 13
6650 Homburg-Einöd

Dr. med.
Klink, Hans-Joachim
Suederstr. 23
2243 Albersdorf

Dr. med.
Knappe, Götz
Hemmlingstr. 20
7033 Herrenberg

Dr. med.
Kneller, Oswald
Königstr. 132
8510 Fürth
Tel.: 0911/776825
Internist

Dr. med.
Knönagel, H.
Postfach 1220
7893 Jestetten
Tel.: 07745/7866
Allgemeinmed.

Dr. med., Med. Dir.
Knolle, Armin
Am Strande 1 A
2447 Heiligenhafen
Tel.: 04362/1631
Nervenarzt

Dr. med.
Koch, Klaus
an der Ringelshöhe 5
6312 Laubach
Tel.: 06405/1426

Dr. med.
Köhler, Bodo
Prinz-Eugen-Str. 1
7800 Freiburg

Dr. med.
Köhler, Roman
Friedrichstr. 46

7858 Weil/Rhein
Tel.: 07621/71134

Dr. med
Koenen, Gisbert
Saargemünder Str. 93
6600 Saarbrücken 6
Tel.: 0681-851949
Allgemeinmed.
Dr. med.
Kötschau, Karl
Lindenweg 23
8201 Schlossberg/Rosenheim
Tel. 08031/71351
Internist

Dr. med.
Hohl, Philipp
Bisch.-Dirich-Str. 56
6227 Östrich-Winkel 2
Tel. 06723/2441
Allgemeinmed.

Dr. med.
Kohr, Alfons
Freyastr. 36
6800 Mannheim — 31
Tel.: 0621/752216
Allgemeinmed.

Dr. med.
Kolb, Hans
M-Hensold-Str. 24
6330 Wetzlar
Tel.: 06441/42578
Allgemeinmed.

Dr. med. dent.
Konze, Fritz
Soltauer Str. 4
3140 Lüneburg
Tel.: 04131/44112
Zahnarzt

Dr. med.
Koop, Rosina
P 7 / 18
6800 Mannheim — 1
Tel.: 0621/22466

Dr. med.
Korkor, Gabi
Klingsorstr. 111 c
1000 Berlin — 45
Tel.: 030/6256008
Allgemeinmed.

Dr. med.
Kraack, Peter-Jörg
Fregattenstr. 2a
2400 Lübeck-Buntekuh

Dr. med.
Krack, Gerhard
Paul-Ehrlichweg 1
7200 Tuttlingen
Tel.: 07461/3234
Allgemeinmed.

Dr. med.
Krampitz, W.
Viktoriastr. 16
4100 Duisburg — 14
Tel.: 02135/4118
Gynäkologe
Dr. med.
Kranz, Joachim
Bodenseestr. 20
8995 Sigmarszell
Tel.: 08389/324

Dr. med.
Krautz, Günter
AArberstr. 13
8312 Dingolfing

Dr. med.
Krimmel, Margret
Friedrichshaf. Str. 1

8990 Liindau/Bodensee
Tel.: 08382/5216
Allgemeinmed.

Dr. med.
Kroker, Hans
Herm.-Eiler-Str. 6
4477 Twist-Bult

Dr. med.
Kromer, Werner
Neckarstr. 16
6806 Viernheim
Tel.: 06204/3700
HNO-Arzt

Dr. med.
Kroner, Helmut
Karlstr. 16
6660 Zweibrücken
Tel.: 0633/3125
Allgemeinmed.

Dr. med.
Krüger, Gert-Achim
Städt. Krankenhaus
6710 Frankenthal
Te.: 06233/27552
Anästhesie

Dr. med.
Krüger, Max
Sonnenfeldweg 11
8182 Bad Wiessee
Tel.: 08022/81073
Badearzt
Naturhheilverf

Dr. med.
Kuban, Günther
Augustenburgplatz 1
1000 Berlin — 65
Tel.: 030/45052706

Dr. med.
Kühn, Wolfgang
Exerzierplatz 7
2300 Kiel — 1
Tel.: 0431/93380

Dr. med.
Kukwa, Dietrich
Neusser Str. 95
5000 Köln —
Tel.: 0221/730830
Internist

Dr. med.
Kunz, Kurt
Bahnhofstr. 44
5870 Immenstadt
Tel.: 08323/8276

Dr. med.
Ladusch, Erhard
Erlenstr. 19
7298 Lossburg
Tel.: 07446/1448
Allgemeinmed.
Dr. med.
Laetsch, Andreas
Mozartstr. 23
5100 Aachen

Dr. med.
Lagemann, Bernd
Oranienstr. 15
6340 Dillenburg

Dr. med.
Langer, Herbert
v. Stauffenbergstr. 4
7209 Aldingen
Tel.: 07424/85353
Allgemeinmed.

Dr. med.
Langguth, Peter
Memminger Str. 178

7910 Neu-Ulm

Dr. med.
Lau, Manfred
Ringstrasse
7109 Schöntal — 1
Tel.: 07943/666

Dr. med.
Laubach, Ursula
Enzweg 4
5528 Neuerberg/Eifel
Tel.: 06564/2390
Allgemeinmed.

Dr. med.
Lechner, Manfred
Prinzregentenstr. 63
67 Ludwigshafen
Tel.: 0625/521356
Allgemeinmed.

Dr. med.
Leeb, Eva
Posstfach 1320
8788 Bad Brückenau

Dr. med.
von Leitner, Rolf
Arysallee 10
1000 Berlin — 19
Tel.: 030/3040406
Allgemeinmed.

Dr. med.
Leitritz, Michael
Schloßstr. 2
7955 Ochsenhausen
Tel.: 07352/1660

Dr. med.
Lepper, Albert
A.v.-Humboldt-Strasse
5340 Bad Honnef/Rhein
Tel.: 02224/2294
Allgemeinmed.

Dr. med.
Leubner, Manfred
Detterstr. 27
8360 Deggendorf

Dr. med.
Leibich, Joachim
Max-Paller-Weg 9
8036 Herrsching/Ammersee
Tel.: 08152/6381
Allgemeinmed.
Homöopathie

Dr. med.
Lindemann, Herbert
Metzer-Str. 19
2800 Bremen — 1
Tel.: 0421/346464

Dr. med.
Linszner, C-Pter
Bahnhofstr. 92
8032 München-Gräfelfing
Tel.: 089/855182
Allgemeinmed.

Dr. med.
Loebel, Peter
Fuchssiedlung
8900 Augsburg
Tel.: 0821/94903

Dr. med.
Loebmann, Edeltraud
Sachsenstr. 7
6231 Schwalbach/Taunus
Tel.: 06196/3603
Internistin

Dr. med.
Löer, Wennemar F.

Bohmter Str. 17a
4500 Osnabrück
Tel.: 0541/21255
Internist
Naturheilverf.

Dr. med.
Loehr, Karl
Leierhof 8
3000 Hannover — 21

Dr. med.
Lohrmann
Hagenstr. 20
2060 Bad Oldesloe

Dr. med.
Lorentz Sylvia
Kaiserstr. 64
6500 Mainz
Tel.: 06131/21009
Innere Medizin

Dr. med.
van Loy, Boie
Gr.-Wilhelm-Str. 1a
4963 Bad Eilsen
Tel.: 05722/84319
Allgemeinmed.

Dr. med.
Lübben, Hans
Jahnsstr. 10
2900 Oldenburg
Tel.: 0441/051876

Dr. med.
Lueg, Reinhold
Weststr. 35
4720 Beckum
Tel.: 02521/3210
Allgemeinmed.

Dr. med.
Lund, Christa
Markttwiete 6
2407 Bad Schwartau

Dr. med.
Maas, Christian
Elsterweg 19
6348 Herborn
Tel.: 02772/2983
Chirurg

Dr. med.
Maas, Rudolf
Hiddingser Weg 40
4770 Soest

Dr. med.
Mackenrodt, Sigurd
6457 Maintal — 3
Tel.: 06194/61457
Chirurgie

Dr. med.
Mackowiak, Günther
Johannisstr. 84-85
4500 Osnabrück
Tel.: 0541/21022
Gynäkologe

Dr. med.
Magerl, Hermann
Karlstr. 6
8407 Obertraubling

Dr. med.
Mainz, Peter
Norderbergweg
2251 Schobuell

Dr. med.
Marciniak-Himmel, Chr.
Ostwall 51
4150 Krefeld
Tel.: 02151/21866

Dr. med.

Matheis, Karl
Haupstr. 97
6508 Alzey-Weinheim
Tel.: 06731/3322

Dr. med.
Mauch, Walter
Rosspfad 78
4000 Düsseldorf-Wittl.
Tel.: 0211/404621

Dr. med. dent.
Mayer, Alwin
Hubertusstr. 44
8034 Germering-Unterpf. H.
Tel.: 089/8414240
Herddiagnostik
u. — therapie

Dr. med.
Mayer, Eugen C.
Blumenstr. 30
8000 München —
Tel.: 089/2604121
Allgemeinmed.

Dr. med. Meisel Johannes
Wiener Str. 54
6000 Frankfurt - 70
Tel.: 0611/595410
Chirurg

Dr. med.
Menzen, Walter
Krefelder Str. 57
4040 Neuss
Tel.: 02101/28004
FA f. Innere
Krankheiten

Dr. med.
Merkel, Max
Lämmerstr. 10
8662 Helmbrechts/Ofr.
Tel.: 09252/241
Allgemeinmed.
Homöopathie

Dr. med.
Merzbach, Rolf J.
Am Lemmchen 31 b
6500 Mainz-Mombach
Tel.: 06131/68 30 00
Allgemeinmed.
Naturheilverf.

Dr. med.
Merzdorf, Erhard
Alte Steige 50
7547 Wildbad
Naturheilverf.

Dr. med.
Meyer, Fritz
v.-Staffhorst-Str. 5
2812 Hoya
Tel.: 04251/2424
Allgemeinmed.

Dr. med.
Meyer-König, Peter
Kreutzerstr. 15
7790 Messkirch

Dr. med.
Mieth-Leichsenring,
Gudrun
Wormersdorfer Str. 42
5308 Reinbach

Dr. med.
Milz. Frank
Hopfenstr. 9
8940 Memmingen
Innere Medizin

Dr. med.
Mink, Erich
Schützenstr. 16

6330 Wetzlar
Tel.: 06441/46645
Gynäkologe

Dr. med.
Möllenbrink, Magna
Zum Kortenrott 47
5750 Menden - 2
Tel.: 02373/81233
Innere Medizin
Arb. Med., Ozonth.
Neuraltherapie

Dr. med.
Mödlinger, Helm, Wolfg.
Grunewaldstr. 57
1000 Berlin — 62
Tel.: 030/7811744
Naturheilverf.

Dr. med.
Molck, Jürgen
Bahnhofstr. 1
2323 Ascheberg

Dr. med.
Montag
Fürstengartenstr. 6
4930 Detmold
Tel.: 05231/24426

Dr. med.
Mpliatis, Kornilios
Lessingstr. 17
7831 Emmendingen

Dr. med.
Mücke, Hans-Günther
Neustadt 463
8300 Landshut
Tel.: 0871/21332
Allgemeinmed.
Naturheilverf.

Dr. med.

Müller, Herbert
Händelstr. 11
2960 Aurich
Tel.: 04941/10041

Müller, Toni
Zur Siebent 4
6640 Merzig
Tel.: 06861/6100
Zahnarzt

Dr. med.
Müller, Wolfgang
Gartenstr. 4
7517 Waldbronn
Tel.: 07243/61309
Homöopathie

Dr. med.
Mues, Rolf
Schleißheimer Str. 130
8000 München — 40

Dr. med.
Naji, Razzak,
Dammerstr. 11
4050 Mönchengladbach

Dr. med.
Nashat, Behzad
Busseallee 37
1000 Berlin — 37

Dr. med.
Naman, Fuad
Neuer Weg 1a
2358 Kaltenkirchen

Dr. med.
Nawrocki, Werner Ch.
Landvogtstr. 4
6000 Frankfurt/Main
Tel.: 0611/558989
Allgemeinmed.

Dr. med.
Nehus, Heinrich
Parkstr. 32 a
2940 Wilhelmshaven
Tel.: 04421/41468
Internist

Dr. med. Netschert, Ruprecht
Heinrichstr. 3
4690 Herne i. W.
Tel.: 02323/43069
Allgemeinmed.
Homöopathie

Dr. med.
Neu, Ingo-S.
Mozartstr. 9
7032 Sindelfingen
Internist

Dr. med.
Neuhäusser, Paul
Schumacherring 21
8000 Müchen — 83
Tel. 089/7146333
Allgemeinmed. u
Zahnarzt

Dr. med.
Neumann-Schönwetter
Neuer Weg 412980 Norden
Tel.: 04931/2343
Allgemeinmed.

Dr. med.
Niemann, Gerhard
Sandstr. 151
5900 Siegen
Tel.: 0271/4133

Dr. med.
Ninnemann, Siegfried
Feldstr. 2
5905 Freudenb.-Niederndorf
Tel.: 02734/6500
Allgemeinmed.

Dr. med.
Nippels, Peter
Schwanenbuschstr. 107
4300 Essen-Huttrop
Tel.: 0201/289081
Innere Medizin

Dr. med.
Nitsche, Christa
Siegfried-Str. 32
6949 Gras-Ellenbach
Tel.: 06207/5293
Pädiatrie

Dr. med.
Nürnberger, Ernst
Senserstr. 2
8031 Neu-Esting
Tel.: 089/356589
Allgemeinmed.

Dr. med.
Nyncke, Heinz
Ölmühlweg
6240 Königstein
Tel.: 06174/5409

Dr. med. Oberdiek, Heinz
Haupstr. 96
7590 Achern
Tel.: 07841/5520
Gynäkologe

Dr. med., Dr. med. dent.
Ochmann, Fritz
Gartenstr. 43
3400 Göttingen
Tel.: 0551/42713

Dr. med.
Ohlen, Barbara
Berliner Allee 40 A

2000 Norderstedt

Dr. med.
Ohlen, Christian-
Holger
Herold-Center
2000 Norderstadt 40 A

Dr. med.
Ohler, Irmgard
Hirschgartenallee 35a
8000 München — 19

Dr. med.
Ohme, A.
Sonnesntr. 19/II
8000 München — 2

Dr. med. Ohwerk, Sebastian
Gunkelsrainstr. 8a
8755 Alzenau/Ufr.
Tel.: 06023/390
Allgemeinmed.

Dr. med.
Orbach, Heinz
Nixhütter Weg 13
4040 Neuss-1
Tel.: 02101/24484
Chirurg

Dr. med.
Ortner, Thomas
Effner Str. 42
8000 München - 81
Tel.: 089/980074

Dr. med.
Ostheide, H.
Am Anger 24
4930 Detmold

Dr. med.
Oszvald, Georg-V.
Tituscorso 2-4
6000 Frankfurt-Nordwestzen.
Tel.: 0611/578267

Dr. med.
Oszvald-Willems, Rita
Tituscorso 2-4
6000 Frankfurt-Nordwestzen.
Tel.: 0611/578267

Dr. med. dent.
Oto, Karl-Heinz
K.-Wilhelm-Ring 2
6500 Mainz
Tel.: 06131/677240
Zahnarzt

Dr. med.
Oveloeper, Arnold
Am Hollemann 25
5790 Brilon
Tel.: 02961/1289

Dr. med.
Owander, Anneliese
Steinhartstr. 7
7750 Konstanz
Tel.: 07531/74647
Allgemeinmed.

Dr. med.
Penn, Hans-Hoachim
Am Bisekeberg 6
7730 Villingen
Internist

Dr. med.
Peuss, Werner
Soetkamp 10
4400 Münster i.W.
Tel. 0251/81922
Allgemeinmed.

Dr. med.
Pfeil, Manfred
Bahnhofstr. 7

6682 Ottweiler

Dr. med.
Pfob, Helmut
Bahnhofstr. 21
8875 Offingen
Tel.: 08224/1311
Allgemeinmed.
Allergologie-
Naturheilver

Dr, med.
Pfundstein, Emil
E.-Kirchner-Str. 16
6200 Wiesbaden
Tel.: 06121/66498
Allgemeinmed.

Dr. med.
Piotrowski, Heinz
Nach den Bülten 62
4950 Minden/Westf.
Tel.: 0571/52989
Allgemeinmed.
Naturheilver.
Dr. med.
Pischel, Walter
Schifferstr. 21
2800 Bremen
Tel.: 0421/383936
Internist

Dr. med.
Pless, Hans-Joachim
Oberwall 41
5600 Wuppertal
Tel.: 0202/622344
Allgemeinmed.

Dr. med.
Pleuse, Gerhard
Am Markt 11
2800 Bremen
Tel.: 0421/327636
Hautarzt

Dr. med.
Plueckthun
S.-Charl.-Str. 57-58
1000 Berlin - 19
Tel.: 030/321 1919
Neural-Homon-
Akupunktur

Dr. med.
Polmann, Regina
Kaiserstr. 32
7100 Heilbronn
Allgemeinmed.
Naturheilverf.

Dr. med.
Portmann, Heinrich
Georg-Voight-Str. 19
6000 Frankfurt/Main
Tel.: 0611/776262
Allgemeinmed.
Dr. med.
Prekajski, Milos
Heidefeld 9
3014 Laatzen - 1
Neurologie und
Psychiatrie

Dr. med. dent.
Presting, Liselotte
Ortelsburger Allee 4
1000 Berlin - 19
Zahnärztin

Dr. med.
Preusser, Wilhelm
Reichenbachstr. 6
8200 Rosenheim
Tel.: 08031/37558
Kurarzt
Naturheilverf.

Dr. med.
Prinz, Joachim

Grosse Allee 28
3458 Arolsen
Tel.: 05691/1601
Internist

Dr. med.
Radtke, Peter-Wilhelm
Örlinghauser Str. 6
4902 Bad Salzuflen -1

Dr. med.
Rätzel, Joachim
Untere Nabburger Str. 38
8450 Amberg

Dr. med.
Ramb, H. G.
Kurze Str. 8
4830 Gütersloh
Tel.: 05241/13770
Gynäkologe

Dr. med.
Rapp, Karl
Rosenstr. 6
8000 München - 2
Tel.: 089/261352
Allgemeinmed.
Homöopathie

Dr. med.
Rathert, Helga
Amselweg 4.19
6231 Schwalbach
Tel.: 06196/86012

Dr. med.
Rauh, Erich
Röntgenring 4
8700 Würzburg
Tel.: 0931/12046

Dr. med.
Rehder, Jürgen
Stübeheide 155
2000 Hamburg - 63

Dr. med.
Reichel, Edith
SPiekerhof 6
4400 Münster/Westf.
Tel.: 0251/44001
Nervenärztin

Dr. med.
Reinhardt, Paul
Bergstaffelstr. 23
7000 Stuttgart-Obertürkheim
Tel.: 0711/321151
Internist

Dr. med.
Rendtorff, Gisela
Düvelsbeker Weg 40
2300 Kiel
Tel.: 0431/3331153

Dr. med.
Rhee, Alfred
Hofkamp 140
5600 Wuppertal
Tel.: 0202/454915
Allgemeinmed.

Dr. med.
Rheinländer, Alfred-P.
Hohenstaufenring 8
5000 Köln-1
Tel.: 0221/237770
Allgemeinmed.

Dr. med.
Richter, Hans-Kurt
St. Johnnstr. 10
7770 Überlingen
Tel.: 07551/62259
Kurarzt

Dr. med.
Rilling, Siegfried
Klagenfurter Str. 4

7000 Stuttgart-Feuerbach
0711/851521
Allgemeinmed.

Dr. med.
Ringwald, Hans
Zweibrücker Str. 12
6791 Wallhalben
Tel.: 06375/395
Allgemeinmed.

Dr. med.
Röderer, Gerda
Ottmannshofer Str. 28
7970 Leutkirch
Tel.: 07561/2061

Dr. med.
Rölke, H.W.
Sonnleitenweg 15
8221 Bergen
Tel.: 08662/8565
Allgemeinmed.

Stud. med.
Rippert, Rainer
Walkemühlstr. 61 d
6200 Wiesbaden

Dr. med.
Rödel, Paul
Yorkstr. 84 A
1000 Berlin - 61

Dr. med.
Röpe, Ortrud
Weserstr. 75c
2820 Bremen-Vegesack 70

Dr. med.
Freiherr von Rosen, J.
Schloß-Str. 3
6412 Gersfeld/Rhön
Tel.: 06654/7217
Internist

Dr. med.
Rothdach, Peter
Widenmayerstr. 5
8000 München - 22
Tel.: 089/297 381
Internist

Dr. med.
Rümkorf, Georg
Birkenwed 21
3150 Peine-Schwicheldt-1
Tel.: 05171/52344
Allgemeinmed.

Dr. med.
Rüter, Bodo
Blumenstr. 11
7141 Benningen/Neckar
Allgemeinmed.
Geburtshelfer

Dr. med.
Rütt, Otto-Michael
Im Oertzetal 20
3042 Münster
Allgemeinmed.

Dr. med.
Rust, Karl
Blumenweg 12
2059 Buchen

Dr. med.
Sählоff-Hartwein, L.
Lindenallee 13
6482 Bad Orb
Te.: 06052/2800
Internistin

Dr. med.
Sähloff, Otto
Salzerstr. 55
6482 Bad Orb
Tel.: 06052/2800

Internist
Chefarzt Sanat.
"Sonnenschein"

Dr. med.
Sallam, Salah
Burdiekstr. 13
2200 Elmshorn

Dr. med.
Sasse, Karl August
Boedeckerstr. 73
3000 Hannover-1
Tel.: 0511/667034
Neurologe

Dr. med.
Sauer, Hartmut
Ottobrunner Str. 18
8000 München - 83
Tel.: 089/407194
HNO-Facharzt

Dr. med.
Sauer, Helmut
Rheinstr. 7
7517 Waldbronn-Reichenb.
Tel.: 07243/66022

Dr. med.
Seehase-Grueber, Ch.
Bahnhofstr. 8
5885 Schalksmühle

Dr. med.
Seelig, Rudolf
Sulzer Strasse
7242 Dornhan-1
Tel.: 07455/650
Allgemeinmed.
Chirotherapie
Dr. med.
Derey, Chan Tong
Adlerstr. 17
7072 Heubach
Tel.: 07173/5344

Dr. med.
Seimer, Hans-Rolf
Schulstr. 22
7832 Kenzingen
Tel. 07644/405
HNO-Facharzt

Dr. med.
Siebert, Ernst-Otto
Schachtweg 27
3180 Wolfsburg
Tel.: 05361/13624
Allgemeinmed.

Dr. med.
Siebert, Rudolf
Kastanienallee 20
2900 Oldenburg
Tel.: 0441/72266

Dr. med.
Siegel, Erika
Bauerstr. 27a
8000 München - 40
Tel.: 089/377137
Allgemeinmed.
Toxikologie

Dr. med.
Simon, Annelies
Hallerplatz 10
2000 Hamburg - 13
Tel.: 040/447855
Allgemeinmed.

Dr. med.
Sonnenschein, Peter,
Ostendstr. 161
8500 Nürnberg
Tel.: 0911/571110
Allgemeinmed.
Naturheilverf.

Dr. med.
Souschek, Karl
Franz-Ludwig-Str. 14
8600 Bamberg
Tel.: 0951/22578
Orthopädie

Dr. med.
Spickenbaum, Heinz
Ringstr. 9
4056
Schwalmtal-Amern
Tel. 02163/2220
Allgemeinmed.

Dr. med.
Sprung, Hans-M.
Haupstr. 61
7601 Ortenberg
Tel.: 0781/34388
Allgemeinmed.

Dr. med.
Schäfer, Meinrad
Prinz-Eugen-Str. 1
78000 Freiburg
Tel.: 0761/73871
Allgemeinmed.

Dr. med.
Schäper, Günther
Kaiserwall 6
4350 Recklinghausen
Tel.: 02361/28005
Internist

Dr. med.
Scharrel, Helmut
Am Taebert 14
2082 Moorrege

Dr. med.
Scharrer, Helmut-G.
Adamstr. 8
8500 Nürnberg 20
Tel.: 0911/351221

Dr. med.
von Scheel, Rudolf
H.D. Teichhöfen 2
3430 Witzenhausen - 1

Dr. med.
Schieweck, Sigrid B.
Hauptstr. 110
2941 Horsten
Allgemeinmed.

Dr. med.
Schimpf, Helmut
Kastanienweg 7
5920 Bad Berleburg
Tel.: 02751/7463
Allgemeinmed.
Naturheilverf.

Dr. med.
Schlegel, Georg
Am Sonnenbuch 19
7737 Bad Dürrheim
Tel.: 07726/5711
Kardiologie

Dr. med.
Schmale, Günter
Brabanterstr. 6
5000 Köln -1
Tel.: 0221/246040
Allgemeinmed.

Dr. med. dent.
Schmatzler, Ernst
Holstenstr. 63
2300 Kiel -1
Tel.: 0431/94450
Zahnarzt

Dr. med.
Schmauser, Horst

Lameystr. 30
6800 Mannheim -1
Tel.: 0621/412335
Internist

Dr. med.
Schmeck, Ulrich
Unteres Tor
7777 Salem -1

Dr. med.
Schmid, P.J.
Talstr. 49
6650 Homburg/Saar

Dr. med.
Schmid, Alex
Gröpel. Heerstr. 155
2800 Bremen - 21
Tel.: 0421/251348
Allgemeinmed.

Dr. med.
Schmidt, Jacob
Herz.-Adolf-Str. 14
5430 Montabaur/Westerwald
Tel.: 02602/3855
Allgemeinmed.

Dr. med. dent.
Schmidt, Fred
Haupstr. 37
7340 Ceislingen/Steige
Tel.: 07331/41064
Zahnarzt

Dr. med.
Schmidt, Thassilo
Hamburger Str. 125
2000 Hamburg -76
Tel. 040/2996122
Chirurg
Dr. med.
Schmdt-Dannert, H.
Haupstr. 15
7267 Unterreichenbach
Tel.: 07235/266
Allgemeinmed.

Dr. med.
Schmittner, Josef
Am Luitpoldhain 16
8600 Bamberg
Tel. 0951/2637
Allgemeinmed.

Dr. med.
Schmoll, Dietrich
Schillerstr. 13
7294 Schopfloch
Allgemeinmed.

Dr. med.
Schnabl, Josef
Karolingerstr. 25
8550 Forchheim/Ofr.
Tel.: 09191/2929
Homöopath. Arzt.

Dr. med.
Schnorrenberger,
Claus-C.
Silberbachstr. 10
7800 Freiburg/Breisgau
Tel. 0761/77940
Allgemeinmed.

Dr. med. vet.
Schöbe, Walter
Freudenst. Str. 54
7291 Seewald-Besenfeld
Tel.: 07447/566
Tierarzt

Dr. med.
Schön, Gerhard
Rothenbaum-Chr. 131
2000 Hamburg -13
Tel.: 040/442867
Homöpathie

Dr. med.
Schönberger, Alexius
M.-Luther-Str. 6
7000 Stuttgart - 50
Tel.: 0711/568307
Allgemeinmed.

Dr. med.
Schönian, Siegfried
Rösslbrünnlestr. 1
7512 Rheinstetten -2
Tel.: 07242/888
Gynäkologe

Dr. med.
Scholtz, Gundula
Hohenzollerndamm 5
1000 Berlin -31

Dr. med.
von Schreckenstein P.
Franzikaneerstr. 15
7770 Überlingen

Dr. med.
Schröder, Lucyna
Bahnhofstr. 15
4740 Oelde

Dr. med.
Schrödinger, Ludwig
Landshutter Str. 12
8330 Eggenfelden
Tel.: 08721/1739
Allgemeinmed.

Dr. med.
Schroer, HHanns
Bismarckstr. 6
4200 Oberhausen - 1
Zahnarzt
Dr. med.
Schulte, Karl
Rich.-Wagner-Str. 16
4730 Ahlen
Tel.: 02382/2416

Dr. med.
Schulte, Norbert
K. Schumacherplatz 11/12
4630 Bochum -1
Tel.: 0234/15 866
Neurologie und
Psychiatrie

Dr. med.
Schulte, Wilhelm
Schanzenweg 16
5942 Kirchhundem - 3
Tel.: 02723/2697
Allgemeinmed.

Dr. med.
Schulz-Ruhtenberg,
Scharn 7
4950 Minden

Dr. med.
Schuette Dietrich
Schwartauer Allee 208
2400 Lübeck -1

Dr. med.
Schuberth, Karl
Haupstr. 35
6650 Homburg-Einöd

Dr. med.
Schupfner, Walter
Lehmweg 51 A
2081 Heist

Dr. med.dent.
Schwake, Paul
Luisenstr. 25
4722 Enningerloh
Tel.: 02525/135
Zahnarzt

Dr. med.
Schwarz, Paul
Ecklenstr. 29
7000 Stuttgart - 1
Tel.: 0711/465353
Homöopathie

Dr. med.
Stark, Franz
6741 Rinnthal/Pfalz
Tel.: 06346/2555
Internist

Dr. med.
Staubert, Wilfried
Feldbrunnenstr. 4
2000 Hamburg -13
Tel.: 040/453345
Allgemeinmed.

Dr. med.
Steiner, Helga Charl.
Stiftswald 1
7000 Stuttgart - 80
Tel.: 0711/682121
Internistin

Dr. med.
Steinhöfel, Michael
Marktplatz 6
8160 Miesbach

Dr. med.
Steinmeyer, Jügern
Damm 18
3300 Braunschweig

Dr. med.
Stemplinger, H.
Fr.-Joseph-Str. 10
8000 München - 40
Tel.: 089/395426
Neurologe

Dr. med.
Stern, Paul
Alfred-Welp-Str. 1
3500 Kassel-Oberzwehren
Tel.: 0561/42445
Allgemeinmed

Dr. med.
Sterz, Eberhard
Finkenweg 12
7405 Dettenhausen
Tel.: 07157/62930

Dr. med.
Stiddig, Wolfgang
Am Schützenbühl 1
7798 Pfullendorf

Dr. med.
Stolle, Ingeborg
Seehofstr. 140 D
1000 Berlin - 37

Dr. med.
Strathmann, Hans-
Joachim
Husener Str. 37
4600 Dortmund - 13

Dr. med.
Strothenke, Wilfried
Schweitzer-Str. 26
3750 Stadt Allendorf -1
Tel.: 06428/3913
Allgemeinmed.

Dr. med.
Stuckrad, Horst,
Am See 18
8013 Haar
Tel.: 089/469820
HNO-Facharzt

Dr. med.
Studemund, Hartwig
Dreieckplatz 5

2300 Kiel

Prof. Dr. Dr.
Thielemann
Rubenstr. 28
6000 Frankfurt/Main
Tel.: 0611/637763
Zahnarzt

Dr. med.
Thiessen, Hans
Hauptstr 6
8997 Hergersweiler

Dr. med.
Tilenius, Helmut
von-Vincke-Str. 3
5884 Halver/Westf.
Tel. 02353/2337
Allgemeinmed

Dr. med.
Tilenius, Wilhelm
Bahnhofstr. 2
5884 Halver

Dr. med.
Tilpe, Hubert
Am Stadtpark 39
3388 Bad Harzburg
Tel.: 05322/2540

Dr. med.
Todt, Horst
Bahweg 37
2262 Leck

Dr. med.
Toker, Yilmaz
Parkstr. 11
2250 Husum

Dr. med.
Tramer
Bergstr. 20
6350 Bad Nauheim - 6
Tel.: 06032/4355

Dr. med.
Tresser, Erhard
Kaiserstr. 63
6050 Offenbach
Tel.: 0611/880557
HNO-Facharzt
Naturheilverf.

Dr. med.
Triest, Werner
Mich. Weniger-Str. 12
8050 Freising
Tel.: 08161/65133

Dr. med.
Troltsch, Bustav-
Walter
Gaedechsweg 3
2000 Hamburg - 20
Tel.: 040/4601130
Allgemeinmed.

Dr. med.
Trück, Helmut
Ringstr. 38
7290 Freudenstadt
Tel.: 07441/2650

Dr. med.
Übe, Christa
Rathausplatz 7
7506 Bad Herrenalb
Tel.: 07083/3811

Dr. med.
Ullrich, Gabriele
Oststr. 10
4924 Barntrup

Dr. med.
Ummethum, Hans
2841 Wagenfeld, Kreis Diepholz
Tel.: 05444/350
Allgemeinmed.

Dr. med.
Unruh, Dora
Arnswalderstr. 2a
3050 Wunstorf
Tel.: 05031/73963
Dr. med.
Varro, Joachim
Taubenstr. 22
4000 Düsseldorf
Tel.: 0211/480399
Allgemeinmed.

Dr. med.
Veldet, M.
Innerer Ring 4
6454 Bruchköbel
Tel. 06181/77011
Chirurgie
Allgemeinmed.

Dr. med.
Venohr, Martin-H.
Neubrunnenstr. 10
6500 Mainz
Tel.: 06131/26503
Allgemeinmed.

Dr. med.
Viehweg, Wolfgang
Lange Str. 35
3510 Hann.-Münden
Neurologie
Psychiatrie

Dr. med.
Vill, H.
Memelstr. 22
8520 Erlangen
Tel.: 09131/24296
Internist

Dr. med.
Vogel, Helmut
Zülpicher Str. 355
5000 Köln - 41
Allgemeinmed.

Dr. med.
Voigt, Harald
A. Schliepstein. Tor 4
4902 Bad Salzuflen

Dr. med.
Voss, Dieter
Brehmstr. 9
4000 Düsseldorf
Tel.: 0211/633185
Orthopädie

Dr. med.
Voss, Leo-Walter
Am Scharfen Stein 3
5778 Meschede
Tel.: 0291/1626
Allgemeinmedizin

Dr. med.
Wachter, Kurt
Seestr. 33
8210 Prien/Chiemsee
Tel.: 08051/4673
Allgemeinmed.
Chiropraktik

Dr. med.
von Wagenhoff, Ernst
Am Gutspark 5
2152 Nottensdorf
Allgemeinmed.
Naturheilverf.
Chirotherapie

Dr. med.
Walden, Arno
Glückensteinweg 41a
6380 Bad Homburg
Tel.: 06172/36350
Homöopathie
Naturheilverf.

Dr. med.
Walter, Lothar
Drösslinger Str. 2
8031 Seefeld
Allgemeinmed.

Dr. med.
Wang, Po-Lang
Am Mühlgarten 47
8521 Spardorf
Facharzt für
Hautkrankheiten

Dr. med.
Weber, Claus-Peter
Waschgrabenstr. 17
2430 Neustadt

Dr. med.
Weber, Erich
Bahnhofstr. 55
2854 Loxstedt

Dr. med.
Weber, Thomas
Rastenburger Str. 10
4970 Bad Oeynhausen -1

Weigel, Fritz
Schuberstr. 23
7505 Ettlingen
Tel.: 07243/12298
Zahnarzt

Dr. med.
Weihermann, Dietrich
4000 Düsseldorf

Dr. med.
Weiss, Helmut
Planken P07, 7-8
6800 Mannheim -1
Tel.: 0621/22797, 812312

Dr. med.
Weisser, Eckhard
Haupstr. 54
7016 Gerlingen
Tel.: 07156/21682

Dr. med.
Weisskirchen, Horst
Kreiskrankenhaus
8857 Wertingen

Dr. med.
Welker,Leonhard A.
Bahnhofstr. 16
6747 Annweiler

Dr. med.
Wenke, Armin
Fliednerstr. 76
6200 Wiesb.-Bierstadt
Tel.: 06121/502700
Internist

Dr. med.
Werkmeister, Horst
Virchowstr. 20
4200 Oberhausen
Tel.: 0208/821-1
Rö.-Facharzt

Dr. med.
Werling, Ursula
Vaihinger Str. 20 Ärztehaus
7000 Stuttgart -80
Tel.: 0711/713099

Dr. med.
Werner, Arndt
Markstr. 18
3056 Rehburg-Loccum 2
Tel.: 05766/722
Allgemeinmed.

Dr. med.
Werner, Heinz

Am Ortfelde 51
3001 Isernhagen
Tel.: 0511/735454

Dr. med.
Wesch, Gerhard
Birkenstr. 6
6945 Hirschberg-Grossachs

Dr. med.
Wey, Michael
Laufbachstr. 38
7592 Lauf/Ortenau
Tel.: 07841/1444
Allgemeinmed.

Dr. med.
von Wiedebach-Nostitz
Beetzstr. 7
8000 München -80
Tel.: 089/472307

Dr. med.
Wiegers, Reinhard
Schwartauer Allee 7-9
2400 Lübeck

Dr. med.
Wiertz, Hans
Lerchenweg 8
4132 Kamp Litfort
Tel.: 02842/4413
Frauenheilkunde

Dr. med.
Wiese, Olaf
Saarbrücker Str. 266
6602 Saarbrücken-Dudweiler
Tel.: 06897/7021
Internist

Dr. med.
Wietfeld, Klaus
Langenbergstr, 46a
4901 Bad Salzuflen
Tel.: 05222/61282

Dr. med.
Winter, Charlotte
Wilhelmstr. 76
6050 Offenbach
Tel.: -611/855468
Kinderärztin

Dr. med.
Witzig, Manfred
Friesenstr. 54
7140 Ludwigsburg
Tel.: 07141/86715
Homöpathie

Dr. med.
Wohlmann, Heiner
Ludwigstr. 48
8100 Garmisch-Partenkirchen
Tel.: 08821/3740
Pädiatrie

Dr. med.
Woitke, Horst
Kirchplatz 17
8370 Regen
Tel.: 09921/674
Allgemeinmed.

Dr. med.
Wohlfahart, Petra
Eppendorfer Weg 159
2000 Hamburg -20

Dr. med.
Wolf, Siegfried-Helm.
Postfach 1660
3590 Bad Wildungen
Tel.: 05621/2001
Kurarzt

Dr. med.
Wulff, Jan-C.

Oldesloer Str. 2
2061 Sülfeld

Dr. med.
Zilly, Arnold
Markstr. 4
5450 Neuwied

Dr. med.
Zipperlen, Irmengard
Uhlandstr. 6
7400 Tübingen
Tel.: 07071/31895
Allgemeinmed.

Dr. med.
Zürn, Ingo-Frithof
Dorf 79 A
7611 Nordrach

Unsere Gesellschaft gehört an die Österreichische medizinische Gesellschaft für Neuraltherapie nach Huneke — Regulationsforschung

Vorstandschaft:

1. Vorsitzender: Herr Prim. Dr. Hergert Brand
Simmeringer Haupstr. 147/9
A-1030 Wien

2. Vorsitzender:
Herr Dr. Christian Herz
Herzog-Stefan-Str. 1
A-6330 Kufstein

Kassier:
Frau Dr. Linda Kluger
Blaslgasse 3
A-1180 Wien

Schriftführer:
Herr Dr. Winfried Muhri
Wastlergasse 7
A-8010 Graz

Dr. med.
Aboufazeli, Housang
Wallastr. 174
A-5671 Bruck an der Glocknerstrasse
Tel.: 06545/477
Allgemeinmed.

Dr. med.
Adam, Christian
Reichensteinstr. 26
A-8793 Trofaich

Dr. med.
Adam, Gabriel
Reichensteinstr. 26
A-8793 Trofaiach

Dr. med.
Adamis, Sotiris
Gumpendorfer Str. 104
A-1060 Wien

Dr. med.
Ader, Harold J.
Währinger Gürtel 74-76
A-1090 Wien
Tel.: 0222/301677
FA für Kinder

Dr. med.
Anderwald, Christian
Lilienthalgasse 29
8020 graz
Tel.: 0316/53616
Allgemeinmed.

Dr. med.
Antretter, Karlheinz
Schwarzstr. 46
5020 Salzburg
Tel.: 06222/73974
Allgemeinmed.

Dr. med.
Auer, Max
Aubergstr. 10
A-4040 Linz/Donau
Allgemeinmed.

Dr. med.
Auzinger, Franz
Dr. Thomas-Senn-Strasse
A-4910 Ried

Dr. med.
Bartsch, Gustav
Zahnradbahnstr. 8
A-1190 Wien

Dr. med.
Baselii, Hanni
Treustr. 15/5
A-1200 Wien
Tel.: 0222/35 71 02
Allgemeinmed.

Dr. med.
Battré, Peter
Gesundheitszentrum
A-9082 Maria-Wörth
Allgemeinmed.

Dr. med.
Bayer, Gerhard
Kirchham 65
A-4891 Pondorf

Dr. med.
Belza, Karl
Untere Kirchengasse 2
A-2452 Mannersdorf

Dr. med.
Beran, Rüdiger
Leonhardstr. 100a
A-8010 Graz
Tel.: 0316/65 82 84
Internist

Dr. med.
Berger, Erwin
A-9122 St. Kanzian
Tel.: 04239/480
Allgemeinmed.

Dr. med.
Berger, Harald
Ziergartenstr. 277 b
A-4780 Schärding

Prim. Univ. Doz.
MR Dr. med.
Bergsmann, Otto
Rehabilitations-Zentrum
A-8962 Gröbming
Tel.: 03685/2109
Allgemeinmed.

Dr. med.
Bergsmann, Roswitha
Auhofstr. 37/10
A-1130 Wien

Dr. med.
Bleckenwegner, Wolfg.
5252 Aspach 175

Dr. med.
Blume, Alexander
Paul
Erndtgasse 28/10
A-1180 Wien

Dr. med.
Bochdansky, Thomas
Porzellangasse 22/2/5
A-1090 Wien
phys. Medizin

Dr. med.
Brachinger, Anton
Markt 10
A-3213 Frankenfels

Tel.: 02725/440
Allgemeinmed.

Dr. med.
Brand, Herbert
Simmeringer Hauptstr. 147/9
A-1030 Wien
Tel.: 0222/74 42 40
FA für HNO
Präsident

Dr. med.
Brandl, Ulrich
E. Knappstr. 21
A-6130 Schwaz
Tel.: 05242/30132
Allgemeinmed.

MR. Dr. med.
Braun, Hans
Südtirolerstr. 15
A-6600 Reutte
Tel.: 05672/2598
Allgemeinmed.

Dr. med.
Brettenthaler,
Reiner
Elixhausen 59
A-5020 Salzburg
Tel.: 06222/79 14 27
Allgemeinmed.

Mag. pharm.
Broschek, Herbert
FA GEBRO
A-6391 Fieberbrunn
Tel.: 05354/635

Dr. med.
Brugger, Werner
Postfach 6
A-9400
Wolfsberg
Tel. 04352/3310
Allgemeinmed.

Dr. med.
Brughuber, Franz
Hanriederstr. 14
A-4150 Rohrbach
Tel.: 07289/8171
Allgemeinmed.

Dr. med.
Casati, Manfred
A-2872 Mönichkirchen 18
Tel. 02649/320
Allgemeinmed.

Dr. med.
Cermak, Thomas
Gusenleithnerg. 30/1
A-1140 Wien

Dr. med.
Chalupny, Paul
H. Tremlstr. 2
A-5500 Bischofshofen
Tel.: 06462/2358
Allgemeinmed.

Dr. med.
Chavanne, Harald
Brauhausstr. 11
A-2320 Schwechat

Dr. med.
Clementschitsch, Erika
Hauptplatz 10
A-9500 Villach
Tel.: 04242/27280
Allgemeinmed.

Dr. med.
Cziep-Keile, Liselotte
Höttinger Auffahrt 3
A-6020 Innsbruck
Tel.: 05222/202423
Allgemeinmed.

Dr. med.
Djalili, Mohmmed M.
Siebenstädter Str. 22
A-5020 Salzburg
Tel.: 0622/21 45 53
Allgemeinmed.

Dr. med.
Dorner, Walter
Glasergasse 18/12
A-1090 Wien
Tel.: 0222/31 25 89
Chirurgie

Dr. med.
Dosch, Peter
A-6345 Schwendt b. Kössen
Tel.: 05375/6/29 103
Allgemeinmed.

Dr. med.
Dudczak, Heidelinde
Seb. Kneippg. 5
A-2380 Perchtoldsdorf

Dr. med.
Ebner, Emil
Mayrhausenstr. 30
A-4060 Leonding

Dr. med.
Ecker, Josef
Rainerstr. 21
A-4020 Linz/Donau

Dr. med.
Eder, Christoph
Mitterweg 164
A-6020 Innsbruck

Dr. med.
Eder, Ramon
Grazer Str. 1
A-8480 Mureck

Dr. med.
Egaarter, Erhard
Schillerstr. 8
A-9800 Spittal/Drau
Tel.: 04762/4000
Allgemeinmed.

Dr. med.
Ehrne, Josef
Schützenstr. 24
A-6850 Dornbirn

Dr. med.
Eisner, Helmuth A.
Breitenhilm 230
A-8071 Hausmannsstätten
Tel. 03135/6530
Allgemeinmed.

Prim. Mr. Dr. med.
Emich, Rudolf
Lindengasse 44a
A-1070 WIen IX
Tel.: 0222/93 64 85
Internist

Dr. med.
Empacher, Friedrich
A-4675 Weibern 70
Tel.: 07732/2900
Allgemeinmed.

Dr. med.
Ensat, Erich
Wiener str. 46, Europaplatz
A-8605 Kapfenberg

Dr. med.
Faulhaber, Manfred
Bründlweg 5
A-5760 Saalfelden

Dr. med.

Fehringer, Hermann
Bahnhofstr. 28
A-9020 Klagenfurt
Tel. 04222/82686
Allgemeinmed.

Obersanitätsrat Dr. med.
Fehringer, Walter
A-9530 Bad Bleiberg 94
Allgemeinmed.

MR.
Dr. med.
Feil, Otto
A-8061 St. Radegund b. Graz
Tel. 03132/344
Allgemeinmed.

Dr. med.
Feil, Wolf-Dieter
A-8344 Bad Gleichenberg
Allgemeinmed.

Dr. med.
Fenzl, Elisabeth
Missindorfstr. 26/17
A-1140 Wien
Tel.: 0222/92 67 565
Allgemeinmed.

Dr. med.
Fiala, Walter
Carnerigasse 14
A-8010 Graz
Tel.: 0316/61370
Allgemeinmed.

Dr. med.
Filipovitch, Irene
Johnstr. 13/22
A-1150 Wien
Allgemeinmed.

Dr. med.
Flaschka, Gerhard
Mariagrüneerstr. 93 b/6
Neurochirurgie

Prof. Dr. med.
Fleischhacker, Hanns
Lange Gasse 63
A-1080 WIen XIV
Tel.: 0222/42 0163
Internist

Dr. med.
Freudenberger, Irmgard
Weinrotherg. 4
A-1130 Wien
Tel.: 0222/84 57 532
Innere Medizin

Dr. med.
Fromme, Konrad
Bründlweg 8/312
A-5760 Saalfelden

Dr. med.
Frühmann, Norbert
A-3214 Puchenstuben

Dr. med.
Fuchs, Theodor
Josefstädter STr. 7/15
A-1080 Wien

Dr. med.
Fuchs, Wolfgang
Veitsgraben 320
A-3970 Wietra
Allgemeinmed.

Dr. med.
Gal, Günter
Weintraubeng. 28/1/7
A-1020 Wien
Dr. med.
Gartner, Karl
Billrothstr. 83a
A-1190 Wien

Tel.: 0222/32 21 39
Allgemeinmed.

Dr. med.
Garzarolli, Ulrike
Fernitzer Str. 21
A-8071 Hausmannsstätten
Allgemeinmed.

Dr. med.
Gasser, Klaus
Aglassinger Str. 2
A-5020 Salzburg

Dr. med.
Helou, Issam
Hauptstr. 68
A-8786 Rottenmann

Dr. med.
Hentschel-Winkler, J.
Jagdschloßgasse 40/2/1
A-1130 Wien
Tel.: 0222/84 29 29
Allgemeinmed.

Sanitätsrat Dr. med.
Herz, Christian
Herzog-Stefan-Str. 1
A-6330 Kufstein
Tel.: 05372/3938

Dr. med.
Heumader Max
Griesgasse 3
A-6112 Wattens
Tel.: 05224/2539
Dentist

Dr. med.
Heyn, Walter
Hauptstr. 141
A-9201 Krumpendorf
Tel.: 04229/338
Allgemeinmed.

Dr. med.
Hitzel, Franz
Engerthstr. 224
A-1020 Wien
Tel.: 0222/24 11 66
Allgemeinmed.

Dr. med.
Hochmeister, Edith
Gladbeckstr. 2/2/15
A-2320 Schwechat

Dr. med.
Hock, Gert
Annenheim 14
A-9520 Sattendorf
Tel.: 04248/2298
Allgemeinmed.

Dr. med.
Hodum, Heribert
Feuchterslenbeng. 67/5
A-1100 Wien

Dr. med.
Hofer, Hartmut
Schulstr. 33
A-4061 Pasching

Dr. med.
Holub, Hugo
Färbergasse 1
A-4400 Steyr

Dr med.
Höfinger, Josef
Maria-Theresienstr. 9
A-3100 St. Pölten
Tel.: 02742/64277
Orthopädie

Prof. OMR Dr. med.
Hopfer, Franz
Lederergasse 25/1/3

A-1080 Wien
Tel.: 0222/43 33 97
Zahnarzt

Dr. med.
Hopfer, Gerhard
Lederergasse 25
A-1080 Wien

Dr. med.
Hörtenhuber, Leopold
Hauptstr. 5
A-5162 Obertrum
Tel.: 06219/302
Allgemeinmed.

Dr. med.
Hosseini, Leopoldnie
Blindengasse 30/5
A-1080 Wien
Tel.: 0222/43 08 08
Allgemeinmed.

Dr. med.
Huber, Herbert
Taborstr. 98
A-1020 Wien

Dr. med.
Hübl, Walter
A-5421 Adnet 19
Tel.: 06245/5060
Allgemeinmed.

Dr. med.
Hulla, Heinz
Angerweg 44
A-8650
Kindberg

Dr. med.
Jachimowicz, Norbert
Liechtensteinstr. 101/2
A-1090 Wien

Dr. med.
Jeffrey, Jaccobucci
Erlenstr. 1
A-6370 Kitzbühel
Tel.: 05356/4594
Allgemeinmed.

Dr. med.
Jonas, Gerhard
10. Okt.-Str. 5/1
A-9560 Feldkirchen
Tel.: 04276/2250

Dr. med.
Jonas, Franz
A-3170 Hanfeld
Allgemeinmed.

Dr. med.
Judmaier, Otfried
Obermarkstr. 5
A-6410 Telfs

Dr. med.
Kain, Herbert
Steyrtalstr. 2
A-4523 Heuzeug

Dr. med.
Kalcher, Gernot
Rehab. Zentrum
A-8990 Bad Aussee
Tel.: 06152/2581
Lungen-FA

Dr. med.
Kallab, Issa
Stadlerstr. 5
A-4020 Linz/Donau
Tel.: 0732/418672
Allgemeinmed.

Dr. med.
Kamenski, Gustav
Mannersdorf 144

A-2261 Angern

Dr. med.
Kapper, Alfred
Haydnhof 6
A-7400 Oberwart
Tel.: 03352/8160
Haut-FA

Dr. med.
Karner, Karl
Puschweg 20
A-8053 Graz

Dr. med.
Kerle, Gerhard
A-6322 Unterlangkampfen 36/1
Tel.: 07242/7311
Allgemeinmed.

Dr. med.
Kern, Rudolf
A-3383 Hürm 13
Tel.: 02754/8200
Allgemeinmed.

Dr. med.
Kernbauer, Wolfgang,
Pötzleinsdorfer Str. 194/5/11
A-1180 Wien
Turnusarzt

Dr. med.
Kiblböck, Berthold
Zöchstr. 5
A-4203 Altenberg
Tel.: 07230/451
Allgemeinmed.

Dr. med.
Kindermann, Theodor
Gartenstr. 6
A-4820 Bad Ischl
Internist

Dr. med.
Klinger, Heinz
Heinrichstr. 56
A-8010 Graz

Dr. med.
Kluger, Linda
Blaslgasse 3
A-1180 Wien
Tel.: 0222/471 471
Zahnärztin

Dr. med.
Kogelbauer-Wechtl,
Gabriele
Neubaugasse 44/10
A-1070 Wien
Internistin

Dr. med.
Köhle, Alois
A-6531 Ried, Tirol
Tel.: 05472/276
Allgemeinmed.

Dr. med.
Kolar, Manfred
Aquilin-Hackerstr. 47
A-3106 Spratzern

Dr. med.
Kolb, Klaus
Technikerstr. 3
A-8010 graz.
Tel.: 0316/78 66 33
Chirurgie

Dr. med.
Kölbl, Wolfgang
A-9953 Huben Nr. 32

Dr. med.
Koller, Bernhard
Sonneck 7/3

A-2860 Aspang

Dr. med.
Koller, Leopold
Raiffeisenstr. 119
A-8041 Graz

Dr. med.
Koller, Winfried
A-8243 Pinggau

Dr. med.
König, Georg
Schwindgasse 3
A-1040 Wien
Tel.: 0222/65 85 94
HNO-FA

Dr. med.
Königseder, Jörg
A-4342 Baumgartenberg 80
Tel.: 07269/205 Allgemeinmed.

Dr. med.
Königswieser, Heinz
Mostgasse 11
A-1040

Dr. med.
Konstantopoulos, Uta
Plüddemanngasse 73/110
A-8010 Graz
Tel.: 0316/43 87 33
Allgemeinmed.

Dr. med.
Koren, Otto
A-9562 Himmelberg 44
Tel.: 04276/3102
Allgemeinmed.

Dr. med.
Korinek, Anton
Hauptstr. 32
A-2651 Reichenau

Tel.: 02666/990
Allgemeinmed.

Univ. Doz. Dr. vet.
Kothbauer, Oswald
Am Windberg 2
A-4710 Greiskirchen
Tel.: 07248/438
Tierarzt

Dr. med.
Kozel, Alexander
Kindermanngasse 29
A-8020 Graz

Prof.
Dr. med.
Krause, Walter
Tendlergasse 15
A-1090 Wien
Te.: 0222/43 15 26
Anatomie

Dr. med.
Krifter, Rolf
A-8443 Gleinstätten 8
Tel.: 03457/212
Allgemeinmed.

Dr. med.
Krötlinger, Michael
Ebnerstr. 30
A-3160 Traisen
Tel.: 02762/2507
Allgemeinmed.

Dr. med.
Kronsteiner, Maria
Friedrich-Schmidt-Pl. 4
A-1080 Wien

Dr. med.
Kubat, Harald
Hagau 245
A-6230 Brixlegg

Dr. med.
Kuchner, Renate
Döblinger Hauptstr. 17/5
A-1190 Wien
Tel.: 0222/31 21 24
Allgemeinmed.

Dr. med.
Kurz, Reinhart
A-6344 Walchsse 79
Dr. med.
Lainer, G. Falko
A-5591 Ramingstein 20

Dr. med.
Lanner, Richard
Sauerbruchstr. 56/1
A-6314 Wildschönau
Allgemeinmed.

Dr. med.
Leiner, Günther
Bergstr. 8
A-5630 bad Hofgastein
Tel.& 06432/8489
Internist

OA Dr. med.
Leitner, Endre
Andreas-Hofer-Str. 6
A-6020 Innsbruck
Tel.: 05222/22705
Anästhesie

Dr. med.
Lenart, Oskar
Villacher Str. 4
A-9020 Klagenfurt
Tel.: 04222/85683
HNO-FA

Dr. med.
Lenhard, Gert
Pfarrgasse 5
A-4600 Wels

Dr. med.
Leonhard, Albert
Neubaugasse 29a
A-8020 Graz
Internist

Dr. med.
Lewin-Ritter, Ingrid
Linke Wollzeile 4/2/11
A-1060 Wien
Allgemeinmed.

Dr. med.
Linginger, Richard
A-4090 Engelhartszell 14
Tel.: 07717/203
Allgemeinmed.

Dr. med.
Lindl, Oskar
Hauptstr. 99
A-3021 Pressbaum
Tel.: 02233/2805
Allgemeinmed.

Dr. med.
Linemayr, Günther
Neugebäudestr. 4
A-1110 Wien

Dr. med.
Linnemayr, Jost
A-8911 Admont 214
Tel.: 03613/2177
Allgemeinmed.

Prim. Dr. med.
Linsmayer, Heinrich
Holzplatz 8
A-2620 Naunkirchen
Tel.: 02635/2118
Anästheist

Dr. med.
Lischnig, Heribert
Gratweiner Str. 45
A-8111 Judendorf-Strassengel
Tel.: 03124/2136
Allgemeinmed.

Dr. med.
List, Erwin
Gaswerkstr. 2
A-2000 Stockerau
Tel.: 02266/3247
Allgemeinmed.

Dr. med.
Lutzenberger, Franz
Rosegger-Str. 27
A-8600 Bruck/Mur
Tel.: 03862/51620
Allgemeinmed.

Dr. med.
Maager, Martin
Horagasse 3
A-2500 Baden b. Wien

Dr. med.
Maier, Hans-Albrecht
Reding 52
A-9400 Wolfsberg
Tel.: 04352/4156
Allgemeinmed.

Dr. med.
Massoud, Ghodrat
Hofmeisterstr. 70A
A-2410 Hainburg

Dr. med.
Margula, Wilhelm
Führichg. 4/3
A-1010 Wien
Tel.: 0222/5270 365
Allgemeinmed.

Dr. med.
Marius-Mathiaschitz
Herrengasse 18
A-8010 Graz

Dr. med.
Martys, Heinz
Markus-Sittikusstr. 9
A-5020 Salzburg
Tel.: 06222/76 332
Gynäkologe

Dr. med.
Mayerhofer, Josef
St. Peter-Str. 5
A-4240 Freistadt
Tel.: 07942/2500
Allgemeinmed.

MR
Dr. med.
Mayerhofer, Otto
Beethovengasse 10
A-2700 Wienerneustadt
Tel.: 02622/3180
HNO-FA

Dr. med.
Meckel, Otto
Langegasse 25
A-8010 Graz
Tel.: 0316/63211
Allgemeinmed.

MR Dr. med.
Meissl, Hans
A-4081 Hartkirchen 83
Tel.: 07273/388
Allgemeinmed.

Dr. med.
Meissl, Helmut
Grillparzerstr. 1/8
A-2340 Mödling
Allgemeinmed.

Dr. med.
Moussoulides, Sakis
Anschützgasse 15/A/6
A-1150 Wien
Allgemeinmed.

MR Dr. med.
Muhri, Erich
Wastlergasse 7
A-8010 Graz
Te.: 0316/34-4-68
Allgemeinmed.

OA Dr. med.
Muhri, Winfried
Peterstalstr. 138
A-8042 Graz
FA f. Innere
Medizin

Dr. med.
Müller, Alfred
A-9762 Techendorf 28

Dr. med.
Müller, Ehrentraud
Kaiser-Karl-SStr. 3/15
A-5020 Salzburg
Tel.: 06222/45466
Allgemeinmed.

Dr. med.
Muszi, Horst
Heilbrunn
A-8983 Bad Mitterndorf

Dr. med.
Nebel, Günther
Parkstr. 11
A-8010 Graz
Tel.: 0316/63 75 94
Neurologie

Dr. med.
Nestinger, Josef
Im Haidgattern 17
A-4020 Linz/Donau
Tel.: 0732/80660
Allgemeinmed.

Dr. med.
Netzer, Wilhelm M.
Kirchenplatz 9
A-5630 Bad Hafgastein
Tel.: 06432/509
Allgemeinmed.

Dr. med.
Neumann, Horst
A-8661 Wartberg 277
Tel.: 03858/2357
Allgemeinmed.

Dr. med.
Neumayr, Klaus
Mittergasse 11
A-5760 Saalfelden
Tel.: 06582/2077
Augenarzt

Dr. med.
Nikolow, Boschidar
Patscherstr. 20
A-6080 Igls b. Innsbruck

Prim. Dr. med.
Niessner, Günther

A.ö Krankenhaus
A-4780 Schärding

Dr. med.
Nitsche, Elfriede
Prinz-Eugen-Str. 6
A-1040 Wien

Dr. med.
Noisser, Elfriede
Bergfeld 2
A-2362 Biedermannsdorf

Dr. med.
Obenhuber, Josef
A-4754 Andrichsfurt 48
Allgemeinmed.

MR Dr. med.
Oberhollenzer, Herbert
A-2511 Pfaffstätten
Tel.: 02252/2580
Allgemeinmed.

Dr. med.
Obojes, Alois
Ritten 131
A-6156 Gries am Brenner
Tel.: 05264/241
Allgemeinmed.

Dr. med.
Ortner, Wolfgang
Floriesdorfer Hauptstrasse
A-1210 Wien

Dr. med.
Pachmajer, Uwe
Mitterberg 48
A-8665 Langenwang

Dr. med.
Petricek, Elisabeth
Anton-Bruckner-Gasse 3
A-3400 Klosterneuburg
Tel.: 02243/2871
Zahnärztin

Dr. med.
Petrinsky, Vladimir
Hausgrundweg 10/4/1
A-1220 Wien

Dr. med.
Petritsch, Hans
A-8992 Altaussee 4

Dr. med.
Pfaffenwimmer, Christoph
Goldbacher Str. 58b
A-4400 Steyr

Dr. med.
Pfretschner, Andreas
A-8962 Gröbming 420

Dr. med.
Pichler, Erfried
Sterneckerstr. 10
A-9020 Klagenfurt

Dr. med.
Pichler, Walter
A-8713 St. Stefan 155
Tel.: 03832/2440
Allgemeinmed.

Dr. med.
Pietsch, Walter
A-4822 Bad Goisern
Tel.: 06135/531
Allgemeinmed.

Dr. med.
Piskernik, Edmund
A-3613 Albrechtsberg 53

Dr. med.
Pitrun, Richard
Bernoullistr. 4/20/1
A-1220 Wien

Dr. med.
Pjeta, Otto
A-4652 Steinerkirchen 78
Tel.: 07241/366
Allgemeinmed.

Dr. med.
Plochberger, Elisabeth
Viktor-Christgasse 1/2
A-1050 Wien

Dr. med.
Plötzeneder, Fred
A-6952 Hittiasau 326
Tel.: 05513/202
Allgemeinmed.

Dr. med.
Polak, Vera
Langegasse 34
A-1080 Wien

Dr. med.
Polzer, Oswald
Melicharstr. 15
A-4020 Linz/Donau
Tel.: 0732/52001
Allgemeinmed.

MR
Dr. med.
Pölzl, Josef
Gartenweg 4
A-8940 Liezen
Tel.: 03612/2205
Gynäkologe
Univ.Dozent

Dr. med.
Porges, Paul
Oldenburgstr. 26
A-1232 Wien
Tel. 0222/67 32 30
Anästhesie

Dr. med.
Preschitz, Herbert
Wiedner Hauptstr. 46-47
A-1040 Wien

Dr. med. univ.
Probst, Franz
Wielandgasse 38/1
A-8010 Graz
Tel.: 0316/72 452

Dr. med.
Raunig, Hermann
A-9800 Spittal/Drau

Dr. med.
Rajtora, Erwin
Mühlgasse 3
A-3710 Ziersdorf
Tel.: 02956/205
Allgemeinmed.

Dr. med.
Ravanelli, Oswald
Pradlerstr. 77
A-6020 Innsbruck
Tel.: 0522/42342
Internist

Dr. med.
Rebhandl, Erwin
Marktplatz 43
A-4170 Haslach

Dr. med.
Renner, Doris
Dr. Stumpfstr. 199a
A-6020 Innsbruck

Dr. med.
Resch, Peter
Hauptstr. 56
A-2454 Trautmannsdorf

Dr. med.
Riccabona, Michael
Salzbergstr. 93.
A-6060
Absam

Dr. med.
Riedel, Ludwig
Prolebstr. 52
A-8706 Leoben-Seergraben
Tel.: 03842/3140
Allgemeinmed

Dr. med.
Riedl, Christine
A-5510 Oberndorf 100
Te.: 06272/7108
Allgemeinmed

Dr. med.
Ritzinger, Friedrich
Agnesstr. 15
A-3400 Klosterneuburg
Tel.: 02243/81840
Allgemeinmed.

Dr. med.
Roithinger, Friedrich
A-6365 Kirchberg 160
Tel.: 05357/2851

Dr. med.
Rössler, Rainer
Hirschgraben 12
A-6800 Feldkirch
Tel.: 05522/26735
Internist

Dr. med.
Schachinger, Wolfgang
Raimundstr. 21/25
A-4910 Tied im Innkreis

Dr. med.
Schallenberg, meinhard
Aussergeldstr. 38
A-6700 Bürs
Tel.: 05552/2897
Allgemeinmed.

Dr. med.
Scharfegger, Günther
Roseggerstr. 25
A-8700 Leoben
Tel.: 03842/5335
Allgemeinmed

Dr. med.
Scharfetter, Ilse
Höttinger Auffahrt 1
A-6020 Innsbruck

Dr. med.
Schicka, Georgine
Burggasse 93/6
A-1070 Wien

Dr. med.
Schillerm Norbert
Sechsschimmelgasse 24/8
A-1090 Wien

Dr. med.
Schilling, Roman
A-2102 Hagenbrunn
Tel.: 02262/4167
Allgemeinmed.

Dr. med.
Schindl, Erich
Bundesstr. 59
A-4050 Traun

Dr. med.
Schindler, Herbert
Davidgasse 11/13
A-1100 Wien
Internist

Dr. med.
Schlossbauer, Gerhard
Puchstr. 5
A-4400 Steyr
Tel.: 07252/58133
Allgemeinmed.

Dr. med.
Schmid, Adolf
Waschanger 13
A-9853 gmünd
Tel.: 04764/2411
Allgemeinmed.

Dr. med.
Schmid, Herbert
A-6830 Rankweil

Dr. med.
Schmid, Peter
Wattmanngasse 24/16
A-1130 Wien

Dr. med.
Schmidjell, Monika
Plankenau 136
A-5600 St. Johann
Allgemeinmed.

Dr. med.
Schmidt, Johannes
Delsenbachgasse 7-11
A-1110 Wien

Dr. med.
Schmidt, Karlheinz
Hauptstr. 2 B
A-3820 Raabs/Th.

Dr. med.
Schmiedecker, Karl, jun.
Hartmanngasse 4/6
A-1050 Wien

Dr. med.
Scholter, Erwin
Hauptl. 1
A-2601 Sollenau
Allgemeinmed.

Dr. med.
Scholz, Wilfried
A-9112 Griffen Nr. 94

MR Dr. med.
Schöpf, Josef
Fr.-v. Walchenstr. 21
A-5020 salzburg - Rott
Tel.: 06222/37938
Allgemeinmed.

Dr. med.
Schreiner-Knobloch, Jutta
Adelenweg 9
A-9020 Klagenfurt
Tel.: 04222/81 68 52
Allgemeinmed.

MR Dr. med.
Schuler, Fritz
Bahnhofstr. 49
A-6900 Bregenz
Tel.: 05574/22414
Kinder-FA.

Dr. med.
Schuller, Diethard
Neutorgasse 18
A-5020 Salzburg
Allgemeinmed.

Dr. med.
Schuller, Klaus
Schmeidgasse 14/VI
A-4020 Linz/Donau
Tel.: 0732/237 333

Dr. med.
Schulz, Norbert
Gesh. Zentr.-Golfhotel
A-9082 Mr. Wörth-Dellach

Dr. med.
Schumacher, Ludwig
Bruckerstr. 1
A-6060 Hall/Tirol
Te.: 05223/6711
Allgemeinmed.

Dr. med.
Schwaiger, Adolf
A-3643 Röschitz 60

Dr. med.

Schwaiger, Hans
DOrfstrasse 112
A-5751 Maishofen/Pinzgau
Tel.: 06542/8231
Allgemeinmed.

Dr. med.
Sadegi, Mahmud
Schulgasse 6
A-2401 Fischamend

Dr. med.
Seidl, Friedrich
A-8861 St. Georgen 44
ob Murau

MR Dr. med.
Seifert, Günter
A-4863 Seewalchen

Dr. med.
Seiser, Rolf M.
A-8942 Wörschach

Dr. med.
Sellner, Reinhard
Schönbrunnstr. 252/26
A-1120 Wien

Dr. med.
Semm, Johann
A-4715 Taufkirchen an der
Trattnach

Dr. med.
Sharbin, Hanna
Pollheimerstr. 9
A-4850 Timelkam
Te.: 07672/5250
Allgemeinmed.

Dr. med.
Sheriff, A. Ahmed
Neugasse 1/15
A-1040 Wien

Allgemeinmed.

Dr. med.
Skopek, Heidemarie
Nonntaler Hauptstr. 43
A-5020 Salzburg
Allgemeinmed.

Dr. med.
Skrainer, Herbert
Haydngasse 10/4
A-8010 Graz

Dr. med.
Smolnig, Peter
Weinberg 6
A-9133 Miklauzdorf
Allgemeinmed.

Dr. med.
Sommer, Oskar
Linzer Str. 4
A-4470 Enns
Tel.: 07223/2010
Allgemeinmed.

Dr. med.
Soukup, Harald
Villacher Str. 1/II
A-9020 Klagenfurt
Tel.: 04222/86556
Internist

Dr. med.
Soxberger, Michael
Lieblgasse 2/47/7
A-1220 Wien
Tel.: 0222/23 73 83
Allgemeinmed.

Med. Rat Dr. med.
Szatmary, Johann
Donaustadstr. 1
A-1220 Wien
Tel.: 0222/23 25 65

Internist

Prof. Dr. med.
Stacher, Alois
Matznergasse 21/1/7
A-1140 Wien
Tel.: 0222/92 43 79
Internist

Obersanitärsrat
Dr. med.
Stadter, Georg
Europaplatz 7
A-2351 Wiener Neudorf
Tel.: 02236/82206
Allgemeinmed.

Dr, med.
Stanitznig, Robert
Sternbergstr. 4
A-9220 Velden
Tel.: 04274/2510
Allgemeinmed.

Sr. med.
Staudigl, Wolfgang
Hohlfeldergasse 30
A-2103 Langenzersdorf
Tel.: 02244/2394
Allgemeinmed.

Dr. med.
Steinböck, Marianne
Rehab. Zentrum
A-8962 Gröbming

Dr. med.
Steindl, Walter
Leserstr. 6
A-7540 Güssing

Dr. med.
Steiger, Wolfgang
Marktplatz 25
A-3335 Weyer

Dr. med.
Stix, Wolfram
Engerthstr. 150/10/4
A-1020 Wien

Dr. med.
Strauss, Johannes
Kirchenplatz 16
A-4407 Steyr - Dietach
Allgemeinmed.

Dr. med.
Stumvoll, Markus
Getrudplatz 7
A-1180 Wien
Tel.: 0222/42 23 39
Zahnarzt

Dr. med.
Tagwercher, Bernd
Postfach 99
A-6780 Schruns
Tel.: 05556/2666
Allgemeinmed.

Dr. med.
Taute, Christiane
Embelgasse 53
A-1050 Wien

Dr. med.
Thym, Wolfgang
A-6342 Niederndorf 95
Tel.: 5333/2482
Allgemeinmed.

Dr. med.
True, Thomas
Krankenhaus
A-7400 Oberwart

Dr. med.
Trojer, Hans
Joh. Panzlstr. 11
A-9971 Matrei

Tel.: 04875/500
Allgemeinmed.

Dr. med.
Urban, Peter
Punzerstr. 60a
A-3300 Steyr

Dr. med.
Urbanek, Viktor
Wienerstr. 12
A-3100 St. Pölten

Dr. med.
Veber, Josef
Seidengasse 41/42
A-1070 Wien

Primarius
Dr. med.
Voigt, Karl
Anichstr. 27
A-6300 Wörgl
Tel.: 05232/2897
Frauenheilkunde

Dr. med.
Voight, Heinz
Chrobakg. 6/3/19
A-1150 Wien

Dr. med.
Vrba, Herbert
Jörgerstr. 26/4
A-1170 Wien

Dr. med.
Watschinger, Karl
Häuslhofweg 668
AA-5710 Kaprun

OMR Dr. med.
Weber, Karl-Heinz
Raffaltstr. 14
A-8850 Murau

Tel.: 035332/2260
Allgemeinmed.

MR Dr. med
Wechtl, Ernst
Sonneck 1
A-2870 Aspang a. W./N.Ö.
Tel.: 02642/2314
Allgemeinmed.

Dr. med.
Wehle, Franz
A-8144 Haseldorf/Tobelbad

Dr. med.
Weintögl, Gerhard
Marktplatz 15
A-3233 Kilb

Dr. med.
Weitzer, Silvia
Kohlgasse 49/I/6
A-1050 Wien

Dr. med.
Wendler, Eva-Maria
Isoldenweg 6
A-9020 Klagenfurt

Dr. med.
Wenig, Peter
Engerthstr. 249/10
A-1020 Wien

Dr. med.
Wenzel, Gerhard
Grafenhof 34
A-5620 Schwarzach
Tel.: 06415/378
Allgemeinmed.

Dr. med.
Werthmann, Konrad
Plainstr. 69

A-5020 Salzburg

Dr. med.
Wiedergut, Herbert
Liliengasse 1
A-9020 Klagenfurt

Med. Rat Dr. med.
Wiesler, Erwin
Griegstr. 1-3/Stg. 2/5/21
A-1200 Wien
FA f. Zahmed.

Dr. med.
Winkler, Elisabeth
Sportplatzstr. 33
A-4470 Enns
Tel.: 07223/910
Allgemeinmed.

Dr. med.
Winkler, Erwin
Sportplatzstr. 33
A-4470 Enns
Tel.: 07223/4005
Allgemeinmed.

Dr. med.
Winkler, Ernst
NIkelsdorf 130
A-9711 Paternion
Tel. 04245-2383
Allgemeinmed.

Dr. med.
Winkler, Günter
Weiherstr. 3
A-6800 Bregenz

Dr. med.
Wolf, Harry
Mariahilferstr. 28
A-8020 Graz
Allgemeinmed.

Dr. med.
Worda, Wolfgang
Riedgasse 12
A-6020 Innsbruck
Allgemeinmed.

Dr. med.
Wötzer, Gerhard
Peter-Siegmairstr. 39
A-6176 Völs

Dr. med.
Wurst, Gottfried
Wolkersdorfer Str. 3
A-2211 Pillichsdorf

Dr. med.
Yanni, Abed
Simmeringer Hauptstr. 93
A-1110 Wien

Dr. med.
Zambarloukos, Andreas
Ferd. Marklstr. 39
A-4020 Linz/Donau
Tel.: 0732/32504
Allgemeinmed.

Dr. med.
Zerlauth, S.
St. Veiter-Str. 62
A-9020 Klagenfurt

Dr. med.
Ziebart-Schroth, Arno
Wiedner-Hauptstr. 95/6
A-1050 Wien
Tel.: 0222/68 33 14
Internist

Dr. med.
Ziebart-Schroth, Rainer
Kuranstalt
A-9821 Obervellach
Tel.: 04782/555

Allgemeinmed.

Dr. med.
Ziller, Hans
Fischer-von-Erlachstr. 18
A-5020 Salzburg
Tel.: 06222/21 02 73
Allgemeinmed.

Dr. med.
Zeilinger, Peter
Schwarzspanierstr. 15/5
A-1090 Wien
Tel.: 0222/43 76 694
Allgemeinmed.

HUNGARY

Dr. med.
Fröhlich, Eugen
Dobsinai U16
Budapest XII

Dr. med.
Gyula, Fejer
Beketer 3
Tata

Dr. med.
Kovacs, Georg
Vaci-Utca 11b
Budapest - V

Dr. med.
Kovacs, Tubor
Dorog-Krankenhaus
Dorog

Dr. med.
Kuelley, Laszlo
XI, Bartok Béla-ut 34
Budapest

Dr. med.
Lakatos, Maria
Piheno ut 1
Budapest

Dr. med.
Rednik, Tibor
Tata

Dr. med.
Sziraky, Stephan
SZOT-SANATORIUM
Heviz

Dr. med.
Zeley, Josef
Béketér 2
Tata I

ISRAEL

Dr. med.
Ariely, Eliahu
Hanasi Ave. 125
Haifa

Dr. med.
Bloch, Ernst
P.O.B. 272
Ramat GAN

Dr. med.
Hameiri, Jizchak
Derech beth Lechem 71
93624 Jerusalem

Dr. med.
Kasher, A.
10, Zecharia St.
Ramat-Chen, Ramat-Gan

Dr. med.
Tauber, Josef
Tschernichow. St. 61
Haifa

ITALY

Dr. med.
Cataldi, Paolo
Str. Leone Fontana 19
I-10133 Torino

Dr. med.
Inzirillo, Salvatore
152 Via Rasella
I-0197 Rom

Dr. med.
Kirchlechner, Othmar
Verdistr. 5
I-39012 Meran

Prof. Dr. med
Lodispoto, Alberto
V. Eleonora Duse 22
I-0197 Rom

Dr. med.
Mattassi, Paul
Via R. di Lauria 6
Milano

Dr. med.
Pavesi, Piergiovanni
Via Garibaldi 73
I-20075 Lodi-Milano

Dr. med.
Susini, Paolo
Viale Roma 12
Massa Centro

KUWAIT

Dr. med.
A.-Razzak Naji
P.O. Box 1494
Safat-Kuwait

Dr. med.
T.-Razzak Naji
P.O. Box 1494
Safat-Kuwait

LUXEMBERG

Dr. med.
Clement, Henri
77. Av. Salentiny
Ettelbruck

MEXICO

Dr. med.
Miguel Lopez Esnaurizar
Avda Oaxaca 7
Mexico-City

Dr. med.
Flores M. Theresia Sabas
Casas Grandes 287
Mexico City Narvarte

Dr. med.
Honorato
Baltimore 72-10-1 Villa Schmitt
Mexico 18 D.F.
Mexico 18 D.F.
Tel.: 683-01-99

Dr. med.
Schenk Antony R.
Tapach. 7 Villa Calient
Tijuana B.C.

NETHERLANDS

Dr. med.
van den Bos, Antonie
A. Diepenbrockstr. 8
NL-5211 S Hertogenbosch

Dr. med.
Bratel, Sean
Visdonkseweg 30
NL-4707 Pe Roosendaal

Dr. med.
van Brummen, D.J.
Oude Kerkweg 6A
NL-1251 NZ Laren NH

Dr. med.
van Bussel, R.G.
Ketzersgracht 759
NL-1018 Amsterdam
Dr. med.
Crol, J.B.
S-Gravenweg 629
NL-3065 SC Rotterdam

Dr. med.
Frey, Rosemarie
Plantage Parklaan 24
NL-1018 SV Amsterdam

Dr. med.
Hoekstra-Gelder, A.
Stadhouderslaan 3
Ermelo

Dr. med.
Kleinepier, Pieter
Fr. Den Hollanderlaan 2
NL-3600 Goes
Homöopathie

Dr. med.
Lamers, Harry J.
K. Aldenghoorstr. 6
Roermond
Allgemeinmed.

Dr. med.
Meessen, Hubertus-Leonhard
Broekhem
Valkenburg

Dr. med.
van der Molen, C.
Herenlaan 1
NL-1971 JS Ijmuiden

Dr. med.
van Montfort, Johannes
Grote Gracht 86
NL-6211 SZ Maastricht

Dr. med.
Oldenstam, R.A.
Putten

Dr. med.
Sormani, T. Vonk
Ds. Sandernslaan 25
NL-3732 Es de Bilt

Dr. med.
Stiekema, J.
Walstraat 19
NL-5011 NR Zwolle

Dr. med.
Verploegh, H.
Patijnweg 40
NL-4461 LR-Goes
Neurologe
Psychiatrie

Dr. med.
Hindrik de Jonge
Warandelaan 30
Oosterhout

Dr. med.
Wullink, F.H.
Holenweg 3
NL-7383 RZ Voorst

NIGERIA

Dr. med.
Johnson, J.
27 Thomas Street
Ebute-Metta/Nigeria

NORWAY

Dr. med.
Arild Abrahamsen
N-1523 Svinndal

Dr. med.
Thor Henrik
Falnes
Moksheim
N-5500 Haugesund

Dr. med.
Idar Magne Elvemo
Boks 55
N-9310 Sorreisa

Dr. med.
Seyffarth
Hendrik
Hegdehausgsveien 36
Oslo
Allgemeinmed.

PAKISTAN

Dr. med.
Saify, Z.S.
305 P.I.B. Colony
Karachi

PARAGUAY

Dr. med.
Binder, Theodor
Casilla Coreo 2209
Asuncion/Paraguay

SAUDI-ARABIA

Dr. med.
Dachiel, Hussein
P. Box 8372
Jeddah/Saudi Arabia

SPAIN

Dr. med. Dent.
Adler, Ernesto
Rambla Barnes 18
Lloret de Mar
(Costa Brava)
FA f. Störfeld-diagnose

Dr. med.
I.P. Loy van Adhemar
Casa L.R. Feliz/Plan.
Altea/Alicante

SWEDEN

Dr. med.
Bosse, Günter
Tvoergatan 4
S-29200 Karlshamn

Dr. med.
Kunze, Hans-Dietrich
Fruaengen
Laekarhuseet
Allgemeinmed.

SWITZERLAND

Dr. med.
Achermann, Albert
Obergrundstr. 88
CH-6005 Luzern
Tel.: 041/415151

Dr. med.
Anselmi, Gerhart
CH-6549 Castaneda/GR

Dr. med.
Balkany-Brandeis
Schweiighofstr. 193
CH-8045 Zürich
Rheumatologe

Dr. med.
Bauer, Ernst
Höhwaldweg
CH-7050 Arosa
Neuraltherapie
Akupunktur
Honöopathie

Dr. med.
Beck, A.
Kornhausplatz 7
CH-3011 Bern

Dr. med.
Bircher, Franklin
Theaterstr. 2
CH-8001 Zürich

Dr. med.
Bosshard, Erich
Fabrikstr. 14
CH-3250 Lyss/Kt. Bern
Allgemeinmed.

Dr. med.
Brunner, Ulrich
Rapperswiler Str. 15
CH-8620
Wetzikon

Dr. med.
Christen, Walter
Schulhausstr. 10
CH-3052 Zollikofen
Tel.: 031/572444
Allgemeinmed.

Dr. med.
Ebert, Jende
Celtenstr. 48
CH-8044 Zürich

Dr. med. dent.
Flueler, Berhardo
Via del Sole 2
CH-6600 Muralto
Zahnarzt

Dr. med.
Frischknecht, Cornelia
Buristrasse 12
CH-3006 Bern

Dr. med.
Grob. Michael
Neue Jonastr. 106
CH-8640 Rapperswil

Dr. med.
Guanella, Nicolas
13, Cours D. Bastions
CH-1205 Geneve

Dr. med.
Hasler, Ulrich E.
Oberer Graben 12
CH-9008 St. Gallen
Tel.: 021/222230, 293721
Allgemeinmed.

Dr. med.
Hedinger, Heinz
Rheingasse 10
CH-8434 Kaiserstuhl/ AG
Allgemeinmed.

Dr. med.
Henggeler, Carl
Bahnhofstr. 19
CH-6430 Schwyz
Tel.: 0432/2244
Allgemeinmed.

Dr. med.
Huber, Karl
Marktplatz 11
CH-9100 St. Gallen
Internist

Dr. med.
Keller, Walter
Wunderliistr. 45
CH-8037
Zürich
Allgemeinmed.

Dr. med.
Linden, Ruth
CH. Luting

Dr. med.
Meiosis, Bernhardt
Jurassic. 10
CH. Wetting

Dr. med.
Meiosis Christopher
Gross ZEUS'S
CH. Gruesomeness
Allgemeinmed.

Dr. med.
Müller, Walter
Schulhausstr. 2
CH-6280 Hochhdorf

Dr. med.
Pfister, Fritz-Erwin
Wehntaler Str. 351
CH-8000 Zürich
Allgemeinmed.

Dr. med.
Renfer-Martin, Doris
Albisrieder Str. 166a
CH-003 Zürich
Allgemeinmed.

Dr. med.
Simonett, Benedikt
CH-5262 Frick
Allgemeinmed.

Dr. med.
Specker, Adolf
Rosengartenstr. 4
CH-800 Zürich
Zahnarzt

Dr. med.
Schmid, Gerhard
Sulgeneckstr. 38
CH-3007 Bern

Dr. med.
Stettenbacher, Maria-Anne
Bim Zytglogge 5
CH-3011 Bern

Dr. med.
von Streng, Franz
CH-5620
Bremgarten

Dr. med.
Thalmann, Karl
CH-9428 Luting

Dr. med.
Tillner, Eike-Olaf
CH-4332 Stein-Säckingen
Tel.: 064/631212
Allgemeinmed.

Dr. med.
Urwyhler, Thomas
Bahnhofstr. 95
CH-3232 Jus
Chirurgie

Dr. med.
Vulliemin, Pierre
Av. des Belles-Roches 1
CH-1004 Lausanne
Allgemeinmed.

Dr. med.
Waldvogel, W.

Leonardshalde 2
CH-8001 Zürich
Tel.: 47664
Innere Medizin

Dr. med.
Widmer, Willi
Kunklerstr 18
Ch-8600 Duebendorf
Allgemeinmed.

Dr. med.
Ziegler, Ludwig
Obergrundstr. 69a
CH-6003 Luzern
Zahnmedizin

Dr. med.
Zurfluh, W.
Hengstweid 21
CH-6280 Hochdorf
Allgemeinmed.

YUGOSLAVIA

Dr. med.
Fogarash, Zarko
L. Ribone 37
Pancevo

UNITED STATES OF AMERICA

Alabama

Gus. J. Prosch, Jr., M.D.**
759 Valley Street
Birmingham, AL 35226

Alaska

Robert Rowen, M.D.*
615 East 82nd Avenue, Suite 300
Anchorage, AK 99518

Arizona

Harvey Bigelsen, M.D.
1135 N. Mesa Dr.
Mesa, AZ 85201

California

William Kubitschek, D.O.
1194 Calle Maria
San Marcos, CA 92069

Hanish P. Porzecha, M.D.*
1401 Spanos Court, Suite 101
Modesto, CA 95355

Florida

Alfred S. Massam M.D.*
PO BOX 1328
528 W. Main
Wauchula, FL 33873

Hawaii

Joseph A. Brock, M.D.*
(Retired)
1380 Lusitana, Suite 905
Honolulu, HI 96813

Kansas

Arthur Dowell, M.D.*
501 Mur-len
Olathe, Kansas 66062

Missouri

Edward W. McDonagh, D.O.*
2800-A Kendallwood Pkwy
Kansas City, MO 64119

New Jersey

Gennaro Locvrcio, M.D.
610 Third Ave.
Elizabeth, NJ 07202

New Mexico

Gerald Montgomery, M.D.
P.O. Box CCC
Albuquerque, NM 87196

Ohio

L. Terry Chappell, M.D.*
122 Thurman Street
Bluffton, OH 45817

Tennessee

James A. Carlson, D.O.
509 North Cedar Bluff Road
Knoxville, TN 37923

Texas

John Sessions, D.O.
1609 South Margaret
Kirbyville, TX 75956

Anthony Valdez, M.D.*
1502 Arizona Bldg 6
El Paso, TX 79902

Wisconsin

William J. Faber, D.O.
6529 West Fond du Lac Avenue
Milwaukee, WI 53218

Please send Self Addressed Stamped Envelope to Dr. Faber if you wish information update of practitioners possibly newly trained in your area.

---

* — trained by William J. Faber D.O.

** — does intra-neural therapy

Appendix II

FOOTNOTES FOR CHAPTERS

Footnotes for the Introduction

1. Stiller, Richard. Pain, Why It Hurts, Where It Hurts, When It Hurts. (Nashville, Tennessee: Thomas Nelson, Inc., 1975). p 34.

2. Pollack, Robert L.; Hunt Gerry; and Rosen, Marcia. The Pain-Free Tryptophan Diet. (New York: Warner Books, 1986), p 18.

Footnotes for Chapter One

1. Webster's New Twentieth Century Dictionary of the English Language, Unabridged, second edition. (Cleveland: The World Publishing Co., 1965).

2. Faber, William J.; and Walker, Morton. Pain, Pain Go Away. (Mt. View, CA: Ishi Press International, 1990).

3. Physicians' Desk Reference, 41st edition. (Oradell, NJ: Medical Economics Co., Inc., 1987).

Footnotes for Chapter Two

1. Diamond, John. Your Body Doesn't Lie. (New York: Warner Books, 1980).

2. Faber, William J. Healing Concepts Issue. (Milwaukee, WI: Milwaukee Pain Clinic and Metabolic Research Center, 1990).

Footnotes for Chapter Three

1. Adler, Ernesto. Neural Focal Dentistry. (Houston, Texas: Multi-Discipline Research Foundation, 1984), p. 1.

2. Bresler, David E. and Trubo, Richard. Free Yourself from Pain. (New York: Simon and Schuster, 1979), p. 163.

Footnotes for Chapter Four

1. Dosch, Peter. Manual of Neural Therapy According to Huneke. (Heidelberg, West Germany: Karl F. Haug Verlag GmbH & Co. KG, 1984).

Footnotes for Chapter Five

1. Dosch, Peter. Facts about Neural Therapy According to Huneke. (Heidelberg, West Germany: Karl F. Haug Verlag GmbH & Co., 1985), p. 19.

Footnotes for Chapter Six

1. Selye, Hans. The Stress of Life. (New York: McGraw-Hill Book Co., 1978).

Footnotes for Chapter Seven

1. Diamond, John. Your Body Doesn't Lie. (New York: Warner Books, 1983), p. 32.

2. Urdang Dictionary of Current Medical Terms. (New York: John Wiley & Sons, 1981), p 416.

3. Thie, John F. Touch for Health. (Marina del Rey, California: DeVorss & Co., 1973).

Footnotes for Chapter Eight

1. Gleditsch, Jochen; and Hopfer, Franz. Neural Therapy, Reflex Zones, and Somatotopies. (Carmel Valley, California: The American Academy of Biolgocial Dentistry, 1989), p. 2.

2. Vodak, Paul. Exercise: The Why and the How. (Palo Alto, California: Bull Publishing Co., 1980), p. 31.

3. Sheon, Robert P.; Moskowitz, Roland W.; Goldberg, Victor M.; Hueter, Betty. Coping with Arthritis. (New York: McGraw-Hill Book Co., 1987), pp 42 & 46.

4. "Solving the Riddle of Myofascial Pain." Emergency Medicine June 15, 1990, pp 23-25.

5. "Exercises for Painful Shoulders." Family Practice Recertification, Vol. 12, No. 3. March 1990, p. 57.

6. Humphrey, Dennis. "Flexibility for the Knees." The Physician and Sportsmedicine. Vol. 18, No. 2, February 1990, pp 137 & 138.

Footnotes for Chapter Ten

1. "Report from the Medical Practice: Introduction to Neural Therapy." Biological Therapy. Vol. VII, No. 2, April 1989, pp 43-45.

2. Dosch, Peter. Manual of Neural Therapy According to Huneke. (Heidelberg, West Germany: Karl F. Haug Verlag GmbH & Co., 1984), p. 170.

Footnotes for Chapter Eleven

1. Dosch, Peter. Manual of Neural Therapy According to Huneke. (Heidelberg, West Germany: Karl F. Haug Verlag GmbH & Co., 1984), pp 112-166.

2. Adler, Ernest. Neural Focal Dentistry: Illness Caused by Interference Fields in the Trigeminal. (Houston, TX: Multi-Discipline Research Foundation, 1984).

3. Neuner, Otto. "The Diagnosis and Therapy of Focal and Field Disorders." Focus: A Journal of Bio-Ecological Dental Medicine Utilizing Bio-Cybernetics in Diagnosis and Therapy,
pp 41-51

4. Dosch, Peter. "Interference Fields." Australasian Health and Healing, Vol. 9, No. 2, Feb./Apr. 1990, pp 9-12.

Footnotes for Chapter Twelve

1. Dugas, R.J. "Submission to the Standing Committee of Health & Welfare on the Health Care System & Its Funding by the ACCPM." Townsend Letter for Doctors. 89:913, December 1990.

BOOKS + VIDEO + CASSETTE TAPES

_____ Pain, Pain Go Away — Audio Cassette — 30 min.— $7.00 includes Shipping & Handling.

_____ Pain, Pain Go Away — 330 page book on reconstructive therapy @ $12.95 + $2.05 Shipping & Handling. Wisc. residents add ¢75 tax ($15.75 total).

_____ Pain, Pain Go Away — Video. 50 minute tape with discussions on reconstruction therapy. $39.95 + $3.00 Shipping & Handling. Wisc. residents add $2.37 tax ($45.32 total). 5 free booklets with purchase.

_____ Instant Pain Relief Video — 55 minute video discusses this revolutionary technology to restore chronic nerve and disability instantly. Specify VHS or Beta.
$390.95 + $3.00 Shipping & Handling. Wisc. residents add $2.37 tax. (45.32 total). 5 free booklets with purchase. (Release 6/1/91)

_____ Instant Pain Relief — 370 page book on neural-fascial therapy @ $12.95 + 2.05 Shipping & Handling. Wisc. residents add 75¢ tax $15.75 total).

Make Check payable or Money Order payable to:
Milwaukee Pain Clinic

MasterCard #____________________ Exp. Date______________

VISA #___________________________ Exp. Date_____________

____
Authorized Signature

Credit card phone orders: 8 am to 4:30 Mon-Friday.
414-464-7680.

Milwaukee Pain Clinic
& Metabolic Research Center
6529 W. Fond du Lac Ave
Milwaukee, WI 53218

BOOKS + VIDEO + CASSETTE TAPES

_____ Pain, Pain Go Away — Audio Cassette — 30 min .— $7.00 includes Shipping & Handling.

_____ Pain, Pain Go Away — 330 page book on reconstructive therapy @ $12.95 + $2.05 Shipping & Handling. Wisc. residents add ¢75 tax ($15.75 total).

_____ Pain, Pain Go Away — Video. 50 minute tape with discussions on reconstruction therapy. $39.95 + $3.00 Shipping & Handling. Wisc. residents add $2.37 tax ($45.32 total). 5 free booklets with purchase.

_____ Instant Pain Relief Video — 55 minute video discusses this revolutionary technology to restore chronic nerve and disability instantly. Specify VHS or Beta.
$390.95 + $3.00 Shipping & Handling. Wisc. residents add $2.37 tax. (45.32 total). 5 free booklets with purchase. (Release 6/1/91)

_____ Instant Pain Relief — 370 page book on neural-fascial therapy @ $12.95 + 2.05 Shipping & Handling. Wisc. residents add 75¢ tax $15.75 total).

Make Check payable or Money Order payable to:
Milwaukee Pain Clinic

MasterCard #_________________ Exp. Date____________

VISA #________________________ Exp. Date___________

____
Authorized Signature

Credit card phone orders: 8 am to 4:30 Mon-Friday.
414-464-7680.

Milwaukee Pain Clinic
& Metabolic Research Center
6529 W. Fond du Lac Ave
Milwaukee, WI 53218

BOOKS + VIDEO + CASSETTE TAPES

_____ Pain, Pain Go Away — Audio Cassette — 30 min .— $7.00 includes Shipping & Handling.

_____ Pain, Pain Go Away — 330 page book on reconstructive therapy @ $12.95 + $2.05 Shipping & Handling. Wisc. residents add ¢75 tax ($15.75 total).

_____ Pain, Pain Go Away — Video. 50 minute tape with discussions on reconstruction therapy. $39.95 + $3.00 Shipping & Handling. Wisc. residents add $2.37 tax ($45.32 total). 5 free booklets with purchase.

_____ Instant Pain Relief Video — 55 minute video discusses this revolutionary technology to restore chronic nerve and disability instantly. Specify VHS or Beta.
$390.95 + $3.00 Shipping & Handling. Wisc. residents add $2.37 tax. (45.32 total). 5 free booklets with purchase. (Release 6/1/91)

_____ Instant Pain Relief — 370 page book on neural-fascial therapy @ $12.95 + 2.05 Shipping & Handling. Wisc. residents add 75¢ tax $15.75 total).

Make Check payable or Money Order payable to:
Milwaukee Pain Clinic

MasterCard #___________________ Exp. Date______________

VISA #__________________________ Exp. Date_____________

____
Authorized Signature

Credit card phone orders: 8 am to 4:30 Mon-Friday.
414-464-7680.

Milwaukee Pain Clinic
& Metabolic Research Center
6529 W. Fond du Lac Ave
Milwaukee, WI 53218

BOOKS + VIDEO + CASSETTE TAPES

_____ Pain, Pain Go Away — Audio Cassette — 30 min.— $7.00 includes Shipping & Handling.

_____ Pain, Pain Go Away — 330 page book on reconstructive therapy @ $12.95 + $2.05 Shipping & Handling. Wisc. residents add ¢75 tax ($15.75 total).

_____ Pain, Pain Go Away — Video. 50 minute tape with discussions on reconstruction therapy. $39.95 + $3.00 Shipping & Handling. Wisc. residents add $2.37 tax ($45.32 total). 5 free booklets with purchase.

_____ Instant Pain Relief Video — 55 minute video discusses this revolutionary technology to restore chronic nerve and disability instantly. Specify VHS or Beta.
$390.95 + $3.00 Shipping & Handling. Wisc. residents add $2.37 tax. (45.32 total). 5 free booklets with purchase. (Release 6/1/91)

_____ Instant Pain Relief — 370 page book on neural-fascial therapy @ $12.95 + 2.05 Shipping & Handling. Wisc. residents add 75¢ tax $15.75 total).

Make Check payable or Money Order payable to:
Milwaukee Pain Clinic

MasterCard #_________________ Exp. Date____________

VISA #______________________ Exp. Date____________

____

Authorized Signature

Credit card phone orders: 8 am to 4:30 Mon-Friday.
414-464-7680.

Milwaukee Pain Clinic
& Metabolic Research Center
6529 W. Fond du Lac Ave
Milwaukee, WI 53218

BOOKS + VIDEO + CASSETTE TAPES

_____ Pain, Pain Go Away — Audio Cassette — 30 min.— $7.00 includes Shipping & Handling.

_____ Pain, Pain Go Away — 330 page book on reconstructive therapy @ $12.95 + $2.05 Shipping & Handling. Wisc. residents add ¢75 tax ($15.75 total).

_____ Pain, Pain Go Away — Video. 50 minute tape with discussions on reconstruction therapy. $39.95 + $3.00 Shipping & Handling. Wisc. residents add $2.37 tax ($45.32 total). 5 free booklets with purchase.

_____ Instant Pain Relief Video — 55 minute video discusses this revolutionary technology to restore chronic nerve and disability instantly. Specify VHS or Beta.
$390.95 + $3.00 Shipping & Handling. Wisc. residents add $2.37 tax. (45.32 total). 5 free booklets with purchase. (Release 6/1/91)

_____ Instant Pain Relief — 370 page book on neural-fascial therapy @ $12.95 + 2.05 Shipping & Handling. Wisc. residents add 75¢ tax $15.75 total).

Make Check payable or Money Order payable to:
Milwaukee Pain Clinic

MasterCard #__________________ Exp. Date_____________

VISA #________________________ Exp. Date____________

____
Authorized Signature

Credit card phone orders: 8 am to 4:30 Mon-Friday.
414-464-7680.

Milwaukee Pain Clinic
& Metabolic Research Center
6529 W. Fond du Lac Ave
Milwaukee, WI 53218

BOOKS + VIDEO + CASSETTE TAPES

_____ Pain, Pain Go Away — Audio Cassette — 30 min .— $7.00 includes Shipping & Handling.

_____ Pain, Pain Go Away — 330 page book on reconstructive therapy @ $12.95 + $2.05 Shipping & Handling. Wisc. residents add ¢75 tax ($15.75 total).

_____ Pain, Pain Go Away — Video. 50 minute tape with discussions on reconstruction therapy. $39.95 + $3.00 Shipping & Handling. Wisc. residents add $2.37 tax ($45.32 total). 5 free booklets with purchase.

_____ Instant Pain Relief Video — 55 minute video discusses this revolutionary technology to restore chronic nerve and disability instantly. Specify VHS or Beta.
$390.95 + $3.00 Shipping & Handling. Wisc. residents add $2.37 tax. (45.32 total). 5 free booklets with purchase. (Release 6/1/91)

_____ Instant Pain Relief — 370 page book on neural-fascial therapy @ $12.95 + 2.05 Shipping & Handling. Wisc. residents add 75¢ tax $15.75 total).

Make Check payable or Money Order payable to:
Milwaukee Pain Clinic

MasterCard #__________________ Exp. Date_____________

VISA #_________________________ Exp. Date____________

____

Authorized Signature

Credit card phone orders: 8 am to 4:30 Mon-Friday.
414-464-7680.

Milwaukee Pain Clinic
& Metabolic Research Center
6529 W. Fond du Lac Ave
Milwaukee, WI 53218